STRATEGIES
for the
C-SECTION MOM

STRATEGIES
for the
C-SECTION MOM

A COMPLETE FITNESS, NUTRITION, AND LIFESTYLE GUIDE

MARY BETH KNIGHT
Founder of Fit Revolution® and Maternal Fitness Expert for
Discovery Health

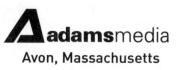
Avon, Massachusetts

Published by
Adams Media, a division of F+W Media, Inc.
57 Littlefield Street, Avon, MA 02322. U.S.A.
www.adamsmedia.com

ISBN 10: 1-4405-0202-1
ISBN 13: 978-1-4405-0202-6
eISBN 10: 1-4405-0737-6
eISBN 13: 978-1-4405-0737-3

Printed in the United States of America.

10   9   8   7   6   5   4   3   2   1

Library of Congress Cataloging-in-Publication Data
Knight, Mary Beth.
Strategies for the C-section mom / Mary Beth Knight.
p. cm.
Includes bibliographical references and index.
ISBN 978-1-4405-0202-6
1. Cesarean section—Popular works. I. Title.
RG761.K65 2010
618.8'6--dc22
2010009949

This publication is designed to provide accurate and authoritative information with regard to the subject matter covered. It is sold with the understanding that the publisher is not engaged in rendering legal, accounting, or other professional advice. If legal advice or other expert assistance is required, the services of a competent professional person should be sought.

—From a *Declaration of Principles* jointly adopted by a Committee of the American Bar Association and a Committee of Publishers and Associations

Many of the designations used by manufacturers and sellers to distinguish their product are claimed as trademarks. Where those designations appear in this book and Adams Media was aware of a trademark claim, the designations have been printed with initial capital letters.

Strategies for the C-Section Mom is intended as a reference volume only. In light of the complex, individual, and specific nature of health conditions, this book is not intended to replace professional medical advice. The ideas, procedures, and suggestions in this book are intended to supplement, not replace, the advice of a trained professional. Consult your physician before adopting the suggestions in this book, as well about any condition that may require diagnosis or medical attention. The author and publisher disclaim any liability arising directly or indirectly from the use of this book.

All photos copyright © StrollerFit powered by mommymuscle. Mary Beth Knight is featured in all exercise photos.

StrollerFit, mommymuscle, restore the core, and Fit as a Family are all registered trademarks of Fit Revolution Inc. The Muscle Bar and Fit Revolution 10-Week Weight Loss Program are registered trademarks of Mary Beth Knight.

This book is available at quantity discounts for bulk purchases.
For information, please call 1-800-289-0963.

CONTENTS

ACKNOWLEDGMENTS

A very special thank you to the doctors of the Seven Hills Women's Health Centers in Cincinnati, Ohio, who graciously gave their time and expertise to this project. The knowledge and passion that this group of doctors, midwives, and nurses possess could fill the pages of hundreds of books on women's health issues. I thank them for opening up their offices, their operating rooms, and their hearts to this book and to helping women. I must also thank them for taking the fear out of C-sections and guiding me through my journey into motherhood. Visit *www.womenshealthcenters.com/womenshealth.html* for more information and wonderful resources for healthy moms and babies.

I would also like to thank my family and friends. Especially my mom who told me as a child that I would be a writer—her intuition proved to be correct! My parents have been wonderful role models my entire life—I am forever thankful for the roots and the wings, the sacrifice and the love.

Also, a huge thank you to Katie Kelly Schmidt, who edited my weekly advice column "Healthy Living" for more than two years and spent countless hours reviewing and editing this book. No doubt her ability to weed through my long-winded thoughts and pull out the vital information has saved readers many hours of precious time! Katie's life as a new mom has often brought new perspective to my writing and without her this book would not have seen the light of day.

And to my husband Eric, through the thick and the thin he has been there and I wouldn't want to ride the emotional rollercoaster of parenthood with anyone else!

FOREWORD

By Dr. Robert Stephens, MD, Obstetrician/Gynecologist,
Seven Hills Women's Health Centers, Cincinnati, Ohio

The rate of cesarean sections in the United States is currently high—very high—and it is continuing to rise. At many delivery centers in the United States, more than 30 percent of births are via C-section, and the rate is continuing to increase. By comparison, when I first started practicing about 25 years ago, the cesarean section rate was about 15 percent. So what has happened between then and now?

A perfect storm of reasons has combined to lead us to our current state of affairs. First of all, doctors are reluctant to take any risks whatsoever when delivering a baby. Physicians feel threatened by the current medical malpractice climate and will recommend a C-section much earlier than in prior years. Also, the use of forceps and vacuum devices to assist with vaginal deliveries has drastically declined in recent years, and younger physicians are not being adequately trained in these techniques, leading to a decrease in vaginal deliveries.

Furthermore, many patients are now conceiving at an older age, going into their pregnancies with medical problems that were far less common in the past. We are now seeing hypertension, diabetes, and obesity on a regular basis. Finally, patients today who have had a cesarean delivery with their first child are reluctant to try a vaginal delivery with their next pregnancy. An attempt at a vaginal delivery after a cesarean section is safe in most cases, with careful supervision in a skilled obstetrical unit. However, most patients are requesting a repeat C-section and declining an attempt at a vaginal delivery. This has exacerbated the problem and has led to an escalation in the number of cesarean deliveries.

Most obstetrical patients trust their doctors. They assume that they are highly skilled and have performed numerous cesarean deliveries in the past. They also expect to encounter no further medical complications after recovering from the operation. However, most patients are uninformed as to the actualities of a cesarean section. They normally have little concept of the surgical procedure itself or of the postoperative recuperation. Most patients go into the procedure expecting to do well, but with little advanced knowledge of what to expect afterward.

The best advice I can remember I learned as a Boy Scout years ago—"always be prepared." Knowing what to expect and planning accordingly lead to excellent outcomes and less stress. This attitude should also extend to patients having a cesarean delivery, which is where Mary Beth Knight can help. In *Strategies for the C-Section Mom,* she expertly breaks down the cesarean process to let you know exactly what is going to happen and how you can expect to feel afterward. This knowledge will lessen your anxiety and help give you a sense of comfort. It will also give you confidence in managing the postoperative recovery period.

Mary Beth's flawless research has led her to create an excellent blueprint for getting through a C-section comfortably and confidently. Not only has she done her homework through extensive anatomical study, but she has also had two C-sections herself and therefore possesses the added benefit of firsthand knowledge. Additionally, she has been present in the operating room for several operations and has seen the procedure from both sides.

What makes *Strategies for the C-Section Mom* unique is that it benefits from Mary Beth's long commitment to fitness and health. She has run a fitness center, written for health journals, contributed to television features on fitness, and hosted a weekly radio program on health and fitness. Her background and expertise give her the perfect opportunity to write a book that is both timely and acutely needed. *Strategies for the C-Section Mom* will make your Cesarean delivery a wonderful experience! Congratulations!

INTRODUCTION

The Unplanned C-Section(s)

Like many women, I had an unexpected C-section. I had found the love of my life, Eric, when I was 35, and we found out we were expecting our first baby shortly after our one-year anniversary. As noted by my doctors, at 37, I was of "advanced maternal age." (I am pretty sure that basically means you are old and this pregnancy thing might not go as smoothly as it would have when you were in your 20s.) Even though I am young at heart and feel 10 years younger than my age, my doctors took every precaution and deemed my pregnancy "high risk" due to the fact that I was over 35. Like every other first-time mom-to-be, I was shocked, curious, and amazed by the whole process. Although scared to death about what labor and delivery would be like, I was convinced that due to my strong body and Pilates-trained abdominal muscles I would have a speedy delivery and recovery. Oh, to be that naïve again! (Being fit and strong does typically shorten both labor and recovery. I, however, am usually the exception to every rule—including this one!)

I went to my obstetrician's office on a Monday, four days past my due date, praying that the doctor was going to tell me I was ready to go. Well, I was sent to the hospital, but it wasn't what I had expected or intended. The fetal nonstress test that had been administered in the office came back with some serious red flags. Very little movement by the baby left my doctor a bit nervous, rightfully so. So off to the hospital my husband and I went. Wouldn't you know it? I must have been a bit dehydrated, and I was carrying a baby who didn't move a muscle while resting. Within an hour, the baby was kicking like crazy! Since the doctor had already administered pitocin, we all decided that stopping this freight train in its tracks was probably not the best move. So we decided to let nature and pitocin take their course, and I assumed that within a few hours there would be a baby! Again, I was as naïve as they come. The first two doses of pitocin did nothing to accelerate the process. In fact it seemed as if the baby had decided to stay right where it was, perfectly happy hibernating like a bear in winter.

Monday came and went—still no baby. But labor did set in! The contractions began sometime Monday night. Ten hours later, and with nothing more in my system than a few Tylenol, I was not any closer to delivering the baby and the contractions were now bearing down on the baby for five to ten minutes at a time and only relaxing for one minute. This was becoming a little too much for both of us. My doctors informed me that after 36 hours of labor, the baby was showing signs of fatigue. I remember Dr. Eric Stamler sitting on the edge of my bed and saying that his preferred plan at this point was to perform a C-section and stop any further stress to the baby. I was shocked, disappointed, nervous, and, again, as naïve as they come.

I had read everything I could about pregnancy and motherhood. I had spent a small fortune on every book, magazine, and Web site club that I found. Yet nothing prepared me for this. My mind started to race: What was going to happen? Would the baby be okay? What happens if I react badly to the anesthetic? This is big time surgery. *It's okay*, I said to myself, *it won't be for a while and I will just get out my computer while I am waiting for surgery, and I will find out what this all means!*

Just then four nurses arrived to prep me for surgery. "Right now?" I asked. "I thought it would be a while before this happened."

"Oh, no," they said. "You'll be meeting that baby face to face in about 15 to 20 minutes."

And just then, it struck me: Nothing ever happens when you are ready for it—not the good stuff in life; not the bad. You just always do the best you can and for some things you get time to prepare and gain knowledge, and other times it's on a wing and a prayer. Say a prayer, I thought; here we go.

I think the most shocking part of it was my lack of control and the sterility of it all. Gone were my birthing plan, and the warm, cheery birthing suite filled with flowers, balloons, and stuffed animals from family and friends. Hello cold, clammy operating room with a slab of metal as my new bed. Suddenly I was wishing that tour of the hospital during my second trimester had made a stop in the operating room. Then perhaps my new digs would not have seemed so harsh. But since no one else in the room with me, not even my husband, seemed surprised by this environment, I soon began to let go of that fear and moved on to the next big surprise: the administration of the nerve block (an injection of anesthetic directly into the nerves or a group of nerves that control sensation from the mid-chest down; it is different from an epidural in that there is no sensation in the legs). There are times when an overactive imagination is good and other times when it is not so good, as I suddenly found myself filled with a surge of emotions, hormones, and painkillers—quite an interesting combination! Convinced that I was not getting enough oxygen, I constantly bugged the anesthesiologist to give me the data on my blood oxygen levels. He was patient and kind, and I soon started to notice my fear of this sterile environment slipping away. I noticed that music was playing, and the nurses all began to introduce themselves, asking if we knew if the baby was a boy or girl, thrilled that they would be joining us for the moment that we would find out which it would be, and suddenly I could breathe. This is not so bad, I thought, they all seem to know exactly what to do, and they must have done this a thousand times before. Women all over this world have C-sections every day, I reminded myself. Four million babies are born in the United States each year, and just over 30 percent of them are via C-section delivery! This will be fine, just fine.

My fears continued to subside as I listened to the surgeon giving his staff directions and informing me of how many minutes were left before we saw our baby. I didn't ask any questions and didn't want to see anything through a mirror. I just listened, squeezed my husband's hand, and felt tears starting to run down my cheeks as I realized the moment that would change me forever was here! Soon after the surgery began it became very apparent to my surgeon that this was the only way this baby was going to be born. He even said, "Mary Beth, this baby was nowhere near the birth canal. We needed this baby to be in Cincinnati and it is way up in Cleveland. I don't think a vaginal delivery would have ever happened." I was relieved to know we did the right thing. "It will be any second now," he said. "And here's the baby."

I looked up but couldn't see much over the drape they had placed just below my chest to maintain the sterile environment (and protect husbands and significant others from seeing more than they need to). My husband's eyes were wide, filling with tears. My throat suddenly had a lump the size of a softball, and more tears were running down my face.

It seemed like five minutes went by before we heard "it's a girl." (We had completely convinced ourselves that it was a boy.) Then I realized John Mayer's song "Daughters" was playing that very moment our daughter was born. As I saw my baby girl for the first time and her daddy held her and snuggled her close to me, the lyrics "mothers be good to your daughters" were floating throughout the room. I suddenly forgot all about my birthing plan that had gone awry. None of that mattered now. And even though my mom didn't get to be in the room to see her namesake enter the world, I was surrounded by a different type of family, a group of people—most of whom I had never met before—who all cared deeply about what transpired in that room. It was not the way I had planned, and not the way nature had intended. But with my bone structure, this is the only way my daughter and/or I would have lived to meet each other. Had I been born a few generations earlier, without the technology and trained surgeons of today, Mazie and I might not have ever had that moment—the moment when you meet face to face and suddenly you know what life is all about. So even though the surgery served up so many fears and certainly took much more recovery than I had planned on, I was so thankful for it. And, to my surprise, it was far less traumatic than I had conjured up in my mind.

Why I Wrote This Book

From the age of 13 to 30 I was overweight—sometimes 15 pounds, but most of the time nearly 50 pounds. At age 30, I quit smoking, started exercising, and cleaned up my eating habits. Within two years, I was 50 pounds lighter and had completed many running races and a few triathlons, even crossing the finish line at Ironman Lake Placid. I dove into fitness as a career with all of my heart and soul. I couldn't believe how much better I felt every day after becoming fit. I was happier, less stressed out, and filled with energy—and, for the first time in my adult life, I felt filled with possibility.

So as a fitness professional who daily seeks out knowledge about the human body, mind, and spirit, I went diving into research when I found out I was pregnant with my first child. I had taken a course in prenatal fitness not too many years earlier so that I could properly train my clients, but now I needed more. Again, I bought every book and certification available to fitness professionals and the general public about prenatal and postnatal fitness. I was immediately struck by the lack of postnatal information. Each book I found had 10 to 12 chapters on exercising while pregnant and then one chapter about what to do after the baby was born. While expecting, I found this odd, but I focused on exercise while pregnant.

Once I had the unplanned C-section, my need for postnatal resources grew exponentially. Why does no one seem to know exactly what happens during a C-section (besides the doctors and the nurses)? Why does exercise after a C-section need to be approached very differently from exercise after a vaginal delivery? And what is safe and effective abdominal training after abdominal surgery? What could I have learned before the surgery that would have helped me recover and deal with the emotions I was now feeling?

Here's what I found: frighteningly little information! Yet more and more moms face C-sections and their aftermath, and need help through the process. It is my hope that this book helps to educate moms on the process, the emotions, and the physical recovery involved in delivering via C-section. I was quite naïve about the process the first time around, which no doubt extended my recovery process. Since you will want a quick and healthy recovery, check out my strategies, which will make your transition into motherhood after major surgery an easier one. This book includes everything from the clothing that will make you more comfortable in the first week after surgery to the type of abdominal training that will zap the low belly sag in no time! In the last few chapters, you will find exercises that will help you return to a prepregnancy state and nutrition that can heal you and give you the energy you need!

Pregnancy and cesarean delivery *do not* have to ruin your body. In fact, you can like your body better! So moms, get ready. It is time to own your body and have it look and feel the way you want it to!

PREPARING FOR SURGERY

The Power of Knowledge

Surprised by my unexpected C-section, shocked by my body's reaction, and wondering if I would ever be the same, I definitely felt my spirits dampened with the delivery of my first child. Before the second, I was determined to find out everything I needed to know in case I needed another C-section. I did, and it made a world of difference. Not only was I able to take a much calmer approach to the surgery, but I also knew how gentle it was to my baby. The first time around, I was filled with fear and was a nervous wreck. I am not sure I can say I enjoyed any of it, until I saw my daughter's face for the first time and heard that beautiful cry. The second time around, even though it was also an emergency C-section, I was confident in the process, knew what would happen to me and to my baby, and was certain I would recover better and faster. During my second pregnancy, I had something called HELLP syndrome (a condition similar to preeclampsia, with additional complications of elevated liver enzyme levels and a low platelet count, which typically presents itself in the last trimester of pregnancy with feelings of extreme fatigue, shortness of breath, and nausea), so I had to deliver five weeks early via C-section again. But the knowledge I had gained gave me a much more confident approach to the surgery and recovery. The delivery went smoothly—Miles Creighton Knight weighed in at 6 pounds, 15 ounces, not bad for a baby who came about five weeks early!—and, within hours, my body started to return to a healthier state. I felt much better immediately and was quite surprised by how much easier things seemed. Knowledge is power and peace of mind. The circumstances surrounding Miles's birth were stressful, yet I was much calmer and as a result enjoyed the process instead of fearing it. This, I realized, is a much better introduction into motherhood!

Although most births are not done via C-section, it is still important for all moms to be aware of what takes place during the surgery and in the first few months following the surgery so that they, too, can be prepared. "The most predictable thing about C-sections—and childbirth in general—is that they're unpredictable," says Dr. William Camann, associate professor of anesthesia at Harvard Medical School. The information contained in this chapter is here for two reasons: to ease your mind and your body and to keep you comfortable—physically, emotionally, and spiritually—as you embark on a speedy recovery!

Planned or Unplanned: Knowledge, Planning, and a Successful Start to Recovery

If you are planning to have a C-section, there are a number of questions you will want to have your doctor answer before the big day. Some of the answers will help to settle your mind before and during the procedure, and others will be helpful during your recovery. While this general information is a start, it is still important that you talk to your own doctor to get information specific to your situation.

What kind of pain medication can I expect?

A regional anesthetic (epidural, spinal, or combined) is the most common type of pain medication used during a C-section, and it allows you to be awake during the surgery. Both an epidural and a spinal block nerve impulses from the lumbar region of the spine, decreasing sensation from the chest down. The local anesthetic used for the spinal or epidural is often accompanied by an opioid or narcotic to provide pain relief both during and after the surgery.

> ## MOM TO MOM: SHOULDER PAIN DURING SURGERY
> With Mazie, I had a strange, shooting pain in my right shoulder during my C-section. Although it turned out to be nothing to worry about, it did hurt and was rather annoying. It turns out it was pain from the air that had entered my body as the abdomen was opened. I am glad that I mentioned it, and I encourage you to discuss any feelings of discomfort or pain you are experiencing. Although I had recurring bouts of upper chest and shoulder pain both during the surgery and the recovery, because I mentioned it as soon as it occurred, the medical team was able to advise me on how to take the proper steps to reduce the pain almost right away. Knowing what was causing the pain comforted my mind and allowed me to focus on the birth. There is a team of people in the operating room to make your delivery as pleasant as possible, so speak up and let them care for you, calm your mind, and make this event as filled with happy memories as possible. ~Mary Beth

What Exactly Will Happen?

Here's a detailed description of exactly what happens when you have an epidural, spinal, or combined. Dr. Bhavani Shankar Kodali, from the Brigham and Women's Hospital in Boston, writes, "The choice of anesthesia is determined by the clinical situation and by your medical condition. The role of your anesthesiologist is to ensure your comfort and safety." In the article, "Obstetric Anesthesia Cesarean Delivery," Dr. Kodali explains the difference approaches to anesthetics and the means by which they are administered:

The spinal cord and the nerves are contained in a sac of cerebrospinal fluid. The space around this sac is the epidural space. . . . Spinal anesthesia involves the injection of numbing medicine directly into the fluid sac. Epidurals involve the injection into the space outside the sac (epidural space). Spinals and epidurals have the same effect (i.e., numbs a large region of the body) because they both involve numbing of the nerves as they branch off the spinal cord. Since the spinal injection is more "direct," the effect is immediate. Spinals are usually the first choice of anesthetic for women who are not in labor but need a Cesarean delivery. Epidural anesthesia takes a little longer to establish desired effect. Because a small tube (catheter) can easily be placed in the epidural space, repeated doses of medicine can be given to maintain anesthesia as long as needed. Epidurals are the primary way of relieving pain in women that request analgesia for labor. A combined spinal-epidural involves a spinal injection followed by the insertion of an epidural catheter. Quick onset can be achieved with the spinal part. Further maintenance of the anesthesia is achieved through the epidural catheter.

Some women who go through labor might eventually require a Cesarean delivery. This can be due to nonurgent factors (labor not progressing), or urgent factors (mother or baby's condition is at risk). If an epidural catheter has been in place and functioning well, most of the time the anesthesiologist can put additional medicine into the catheter to make the numbness adequate for surgery. As with spinal anesthesia, it is normal for the body to feel numb from the lower chest down to the feet. Again, this is considered the right amount of anesthesia to keep you comfortable for the operation.

In cases of emergency C-sections, general anesthesia may be used instead. Administered more quickly, it induces a sleep-like state for the mom-to-be.

The Immediate Effects

While the process of injecting the anesthetic can be a bit alarming, (I haven't met anyone yet who likes needles), have no fear. The anesthesiologist is a pro and likely prepares dozens of patients for surgery most days of the week. I was surprised how quickly the surgery began after the nerve block was administered. The medication does take effect quickly and it does give some peace of mind to know the signs of its effectiveness prior to the onset of surgery. Within moments, you may feel a warm sensation spread through the legs and chest; this is often accompanied by a tingling sensation. Your blood pressure may lower slightly after the drugs have taken effect; if this is the case the warm sensation will be replaced by feeling quite cold. The drop in blood pressure may feel alarming to you, but it happens often and the anesthesiologist is monitoring all your vital signs! Since the anesthetic also numbs your chest, your brain may not recognize the fact that you are breathing normally. Try not to let this lack of proper communication between the brain and the lungs fill you with fear as it did me. These are all typical responses, and again, your every breath is being watched closely. In addition, as long as you are able to talk you are getting the oxygen that you need. It is also very typical for your anesthesiologist to ask you questions about the numbness you feel shortly after it is administered. He or she is simply checking to make sure that the amount given ensures that the only sensations you will feel during the birth are pulling or tugging, and perhaps pressure as your medical team works to deliver the baby.

Possible Reactions

Even though allergic reactions to epidurals and spinals occur infrequently, women do have a 60 percent greater chance of a mildly adverse reaction to narcotics than men do. It is important for you to review your own medical history and make sure that you have not had any adverse effects from the planned medication or related medications in the past. Again, having a conversation with your doctor prior to surgery is a great strategy. Even if you are in the midst of an unplanned C-section and there is little time for preparation, have your partner or a family member review the symptoms of a reaction with a nurse, doctor, or anesthesiologist. While you might not be able to put two and two together shortly after surgery, your support team will have a better view of the overall picture and might recognize it more quickly than you. Besides, all those people who love you and are hovering tend to feel a little less helpless at this point. Here are some typical side effects of an anesthesia:

- Numbness for a number of hours postsurgery (ask for help if getting out of bed!)
- Soreness at site of insertion
- Ringing of the ears
- Shivering
- Anxiety
- Constipation and difficulty urinating
- Headache
- Decreased blood pressure, which can lead to nausea

Atypical side effects that signal an adverse reaction yet are easily treated:

- Skin reaction
- Itching

- Pain at the site of insertion
- Burning
- Slight inflammation
- Nausea
- Vomiting

More serious side effects:

- Difficulty breathing
- Asthma-like symptoms

If these occur, alert a member of the medical staff immediately. Most symptoms can be treated and alleviated rather quickly. The earlier you notice them the less symptomatic you may become!

How long will the procedure take, and will you tell me if it will take longer than you originally planned?

Most standard C-sections take place from start to finish in about an hour. Most of that time is spent prepping you, administering the anesthetic, and then suturing you back up after the delivery. Most of the time, it takes only five minutes from the first incision on the skin to the time the baby is born, and even though the baby comes relatively quickly, it will seem like an eternity before you are in recovery and holding your new baby in your arms.

During my research, thousands of moms in the StrollerFit exercise program across the country were kind enough to participate in a survey. I asked them many questions and learned a lot from them. One question in particular I felt was very important: "What was the one thing you wished you had known before your C-section?" Eighty percent of them answered the same way: "I wish I had known that I wouldn't be able to hold my baby right away." I second their answer. I had no idea that I wouldn't hold Mazie until almost an hour later in recovery. Looking back, I understand why, but at that moment, the moment I had waited so long for, I didn't understand. I wanted to hold that little girl in my arms and let her hear my voice. I wanted to feel her heartbeat, look into her little eyes, and welcome her into this world.

MOM to MOM: MEDICINE ALLERGIES

My first C-section came with an allergic reaction to duramorph, the pain medication that had been administered, which left me covered in hives and welts about six hours after delivering. Talk about miserable—I can remember holding my daughter for the first time and wondering why my faced itched so badly. It was a few more hours before we realized that I was having a bad reaction to the medication and the nurses began to deliver an antihistamine through my IV line. Every four hours a new dose brought some relief, but as the antihistamine began to wear off after two hours, I was left to count down the itching hours by the minute until the next dose of relief.

The hives were huge, and the itching was unlike anything I had ever felt before. All could have been prevented though, had I known to ask! Had I asked, I would have found out that as a child I had a bad reaction to a medication that is "related" to duramorph. Had I done a little more digging, I would have found out that my father has many drug allergies, and I am my father's daughter. You better believe I discussed this with my obstetrical team during my second pregnancy! I was not going to suffer that way again. Dr. Stephens recommended I speak with the hospital's anesthesiologist to formulate a plan for the second go-round. We used another anesthetic, and he also administered the antihistamine shortly after delivery, just in case. The plan worked like a charm—no itching, no hives, and still the same lack of feeling and pain relief! Moral of the story: It pays to know your medical history and to ask questions. ~Mary Beth

My advice for all of you moms to be: Let your partner know that you won't be able to hold your baby until recovery. Ask your partner to make sure to bring your baby close to your face, close enough for you to hear the baby's heart and feel the baby's breath, and close enough for the baby to feel, hear, and see you. Rub your baby's little fingers on your face and your fingers on the baby. You won't have long; the nurses will want to get all the measurements and begin the Apgar tests.

Also, prior to surgery, ask someone on the delivery team to take pictures for you. Your partner will be holding your little bundle of joy and won't have enough hands to take the pictures too.

Don't be afraid to ask your doctor how long he or she expects the procedure to take, and if you find yourself worried during the procedure, put your mind at ease and ask any and all questions that come to mind.

Can I see the operating room ahead of time?

Many moms that I surveyed had never been in an operating room prior to their C-section, and most, including myself, were somewhat shocked by the room itself. If at all possible, ask your physician or hospital if you can take a peek into the operating room. This is a chance for you to alleviate any unnecessary fear you might have. Even if you don't think you will be fearful, hormones and emotions can change your mood drastically! So take the opportunity to check it out ahead of time.

How exactly does your practice conduct a C-section surgery?

There are seven layers of tissue that the doctor must move through to deliver your baby. In a typical, nonemergency C-section, your doctor will make a transverse (horizontal) incision in the skin, the subcutaneous fat, and the fascia (a connective tissue that envelopes like muscle fibers). The incision of the skin layer traditionally occurs at the "bikini line" and is hardly noticeable after healing. He or she will then separate the rectus abdominis (commonly known as the six-pack muscle) by hand and/or instrument. Following the separation of the rectus, a transverse incision will be made into the abdominal peritoneum, a thin, smooth membrane providing protection for the organs, after which the bladder will be temporarily pushed down to allow the doctor access to the uterus.

After a transverse incision in the peritoneum protecting the uterus, a transverse cut into the uterus will allow for the baby to be delivered. Transverse incisions heal faster and often allow for future vaginal deliveries to take place. It is only on rare occasions that a vertical incision is made into the uterus—usually when a larger opening is necessary to deliver the baby. After the incision into the uterus is completed, the amniotic sac is opened and the baby is delivered. It is during the time when the baby is delivered from the uterus that you may feel pressure. Other than this, your experience should be pain-free.

Once your baby is born, the doctor will clamp and cut the umbilical cord. Following the umbilical cord procedures, the placenta will be removed and the doctor will begin to suture the layers disturbed during the procedure.

Do you stitch and approximate all seven layers, or just three layers?

According to Dr. Robert Stephens, MD, obstetrician/gynecologist at Seven Hills Women's Health Centers in Cincinnati, Ohio, there are two courses of actions that obstetric practices choose between for C-section surgery:

1. All seven layers of tissue are sutured or stapled together; or
2. Just three layers, (uterus, fascia, and skin) are sutured.

Dr. Stephens believes that loosely approximating (suturing) *all* of the layers speeds the healing process, and I am thankful that the practice he is a part of follows this lengthier process.

If all seven layers are reconnected, the uterus is stitched first, followed by a loose approximation of the peritoneum. The doctor will return the bladder to its original position, and then loosely approximate the abdominal peritoneum. The doctor will then place loose sutures pulling the rectus abdominis back together, which can help prevent or alleviate diastasis recti (separation of the two halves of the muscle due to the softening of the linea alba).

Second in importance to the closure of the uterus is the stitching of the fascia, which is done meticulously to decrease the risk of hernia.

Next, the doctor loosely stitches the subcutaneous fat layer to prevent dimpling or sinking of this tissue beneath the scar on the skin, and last, he or she places the sutures or staples, closing the skin.

Now, that was not nearly as bad as you might have envisioned, and I can assure you from witnessing two C-section surgeries, it is a beautiful and gentle process.

Ask your physician, even if he or she usually only sutures the three layers, to reattach all seven. I believe—as a result of my research and my knowledge as a fitness professional and a mom who delivered two babies via C-section—that reconnecting all seven layers will speed your healing process.

One more piece of advice: Just for fun, watch your doctor's facial expressions as you ask this question. He or she is sure to be impressed with your knowledge, research, and desire for well-being!

Bags Packed and Ready to Go!

By now, you have most likely read every pregnancy book or magazine and have seen hundreds of lists on what you should plan on packing for the hospital. I did too. A surprise C-section later, and I wish I had packed differently. If you know a C-section is in your not-so-distant future, you'll need to add a few items to your list that will make your hospital stay and trip home more comfortable. If you don't plan on having a C-section and end up surprised, send your partner or a family member home for a few items within a few hours after the surgery so that you too can ease into recovery and your new life as a mom.

Make sure these items are in your bag. . . .

This Book

All the information about the surgery itself, pain medication, pain management, and what to ask your doctor are right here! There is a very small chance that you will remember everything without rereading it for a few days in a row. It is also not a bad idea that those around you read the pain management section of the book. As your support team, they will be looking for ways to aid you in your recovery and to help you transition into motherhood. It will also be helpful as fatigue and pain medication will more than likely impair your ability to recall this information.

The Right Clothes (Especially Underwear and Pants!)

Boy, do I wish I knew then what I know now! Many women will find themselves retaining quite a bit of water postsurgery and are surprised at how swollen the tissue of the abdomen can become in the first days and weeks after surgery. Wishful thinking might lead you to bring a smaller size of pants and underwear with you to the hospital. In reality, the same size as you wore in is the smarter choice for going home. And as much as I hate to say it (and you will hate to hear it), bring a pair of pants that is one size up from the ones you fit into the day you deliver.

> ## MOM to MOM: MESH PANTIES
> I brought my granny panties, but instead stayed in the mesh panties from the hospital for the first few days because my belly was so swollen from surgery that even the granny panties didn't fit well. I actually wore them for a few days at home as well. Moms shouldn't expect to wear nonmaternity pants for a few weeks. I knew I would be swollen but I didn't know that my pants would be tighter leaving the hospital than they were going in! ~Natalie

But there is more to the pants than just size alone.

Pack pants and underwear that are *not* the low-rise style. Odds are, the incision on your skin will be just below your "bikini line." Whether or not you own a bikini or wear one is unimportant; knowing where this incision is made on your body is very important for comfort and healing, both while awake and while sleeping. Low-rise pants, skirts, underwear, and/or pajamas will mostly hit too close to your scar for your liking. Although low-rise maternity clothing might suit you best and be most comfortable during pregnancy, do not count on wearing it during the first week or two postsurgery. Instead, bring clothing that comes up halfway between where you believe your bikini line to be and your navel.

Also, do not plan on wearing anything with a zipper, or any pants, shorts, or skirts that require a belt. Pressure, chaffing, or tightness on the C-section scar will most certainly add to your discomfort. My personal favorite for the first two weeks following a C-section are roll-top yoga-style pants. This style allows you to decide how high or low the top of your pants are and are easy to put on and take off, even when your pain level is higher than you'd like it to be. While drawstring pants did not work well for me, another C-section mom friend of mind found them to work best for her, but she also recommends bringing a size larger than you think you may need. Underwear requires the same thought process, and if I could do it all over again I would say bring on the granny panties or the boy shorts! Again, where the top of the underwear touches your body is important for your comfort, and having your undergarments a little roomy will prove to be much more comfortable than having them a little too tight.

MOM to MOM: GETTING DRESSED POSTSURGERY

After my C-section, I tried to wear maternity yoga pants, thinking that the stretchy waist would be comfortable. But the added pressure on my gas-filled belly made me miserable and I felt better immediately after changing into drawstring pajama pants. A nurse in the hospital gave me the tip to place a pad between my underwear and the incision. That enabled me to wear elastic-waist pants a little sooner. ~Sarah

I will never forget feeling like an overstuffed sausage in the hospital-issued postop underpants. *Yikes!* Not only were they a little snug, but they were also fishnet style. No, the hospital I was in did not supply sexy fishnet; it was more like surgical net underwear that was less than attractive and horribly uncomfortable. My discomfort with the hospital issued undies stemmed from being pumped full of fluids for two days prior to actually delivering and all of that fluid sat right between my hips and thighs for a good while. A friend of mine who delivered twins via C-sections loved them! She said "Wear the mesh undies they give you. Loved those things. Everyone makes fun of them but *wow*! Those were better than my panties for while the stitches were still annoying and rubbing on fabric!" Moral of the story *be prepared* . . . pack your own undies! Pack a few different types and sizes, and three times as many pairs as you think you will need! Your partner and family might think you have gone a little overboard, but you will be comfortable!

Loose-fitting tops, jackets, or button-down shirts are also a great item to pack. Any top that has elastic around the waist can also lead to discomfort.

Pack a pair of comfortable, slip-on shoes that are not slippers! Having aided my mom for a number of months as she recovered from a fall down the steps caused by slippery slippers, I have become a fan of slip-on shoes with real soles, and I tossed all my slippers aside! You will need to get up from your bed within a few hours of your surgery. The nerve block and pain medication will more than likely make you a little unsteady, and the last thing you need is a pair of slippers that could cause more unsteadiness.

By now you probably feel as if you are overthinking this two- to four-day stay in the hospital, but in the end, a little thought goes a long way.

Prepping for Surgery

If you know ahead of time that you are having a C-section, you can begin to prepare yourself before you check into the hospital. If you are anything like me (a little shy when it comes to being naked in front of strangers), a little preparation at home can help make you feel more comfortable. Because the incision takes place at the bikini line, the nurses will shave you' before surgery. I highly recommend doing as much of this at home as possible. Although kindhearted, the nurses might not take as much time or be as gentle as you would be! Girl-to-girl, this can be a difficult thing to do in the last few days before your delivery, but try if you can!

You will be told to arrive at the hospital a number of hours before you are scheduled in the operating room. You will be told to not eat anything beginning at a certain time. Though it may seem like an extra hardship, an empty stomach is necessary for your health and well-being, and it lowers the risk of vomiting and nausea during surgery. Even though you may feel hungry and want to eat, these feelings will pass once the nerve block and pain medication enter your system. Pain medication often slows the metabolism, thus reducing the number of calories you burn even while lying in bed. This process leaves you less hungry and less concerned with food.

You will likely be given an antacid to further suppress nausea and reduce the likelihood of vomiting. This is important for two reasons: one, it is uncomfortable and a little scary to get sick in the operating room, and two, it will lower the risk of pneumonia. Pneumonia is an infection of the lungs that causes the alveoli to fill with fluid, making it difficult to breathe. Major surgery puts you more at risk for pneumonia because of a weakened immune system as well as difficulty coughing, which is the body's first line of defense and the fastest way for your body to rid itself of unwanted particles. Furthermore, the transversus abdominis has a hard time contracting properly post-C-section and it is responsible for deep exhalation, coughing, sneezing, and childbirth. With this muscle incapable of properly assisting in coughing, along with extended bed rest that can lead to fluid and mucus gathering in the lungs postsurgery, your body becomes the perfect place for bacteria to grow. Aspiration pneumonia is a lung infection that can occur from inhaling mouth secretions and stomach contents, which is why it is important to limit the risk of vomiting. An IV will be placed in your arm to aid in keeping you hydrated as well as providing a fast delivery system for pain medication and antinausea medicine if necessary. A catheter will be inserted into your bladder and will remain there typically until the morning after the surgery. Blood pressure and heart rate monitors will be attached prior to the surgery so that constant monitoring of your vital signs can take place prior to, during, and for the first 24 to 48 hours after surgery.

Postsurgery

Once the surgery and suturing are finished, you'll be moved into recovery, where you can finally snuggle with your baby. Most likely, the painkillers administered during surgery are still in full force. Good thing! Expect to spend a few hours in recovery before heading to the room where you'll spend the remainder of your time in the hospital. In postop, nurses will monitor your vital signs, and if you choose to breastfeed you will most likely have your first experience here.

Feeding the Baby Postsurgery

Breastfeeding immediately following a C-section can be a challenge—between the pain medication and your decreased mobility following surgery, you'll need some extra help. So ask the nurses! They can help get the baby into a comfortable position for breast- or bottle-feeding. I found it nearly impossible to use a Boppy or other "feeding" pillow that was supposed to wrap around my abdomen and offer support. For the first few days, using a few regular pillows might keep you the most comfortable. It is also important to think about lower back support, whether this means sitting in a chair that offers support or arranging pillows in such a manner that your spine remain relatively straight. A rounded lower back can compress the lumbar region vertebrae, causing lower back discomfort, and a rounded upper back can lead to shoulder fatigue as well as a stiff and/or sore neck. Since your postural muscles (the ones that help keep your spine straight) are weakened from pregnancy, you may find good posture difficult to achieve without a supportive chair or the aid of pillows. Whenever possible, try to maintain good posture.

In Your Room

Your family, who may have spent hours in the waiting room, will probably be allowed to trickle into the recovery area to see you and the baby as long as you and baby are both doing well, and as long as it is not too disruptive to the other patients in recovery.

After a few hours in recovery, you will be moved to your room, where you will meet the nurses responsible for your care for the next few hours and days. I still remember the names and faces of all the nurses who cared for me after both deliveries. These women and men truly loved their jobs, and I never once recall seeing anything but a smile on their faces.

Gentle Movement to Promote Healing

Actually, the only time that I wasn't completely happy with the nursing team was when they dragged me out of bed for that first postop walk—a dirty job, but someone has to make you do it!

"This has to be a horrible mistake," I thought. "I just had major surgery after 36 hours of labor, and I think I fell asleep maybe 45 minutes ago. It is 2 A.M. This nurse must have the wrong patient. It would be cruel and unusual punishment to make me get out of bed. Surely this is a mistake." But no!

Turns out that getting up and walking around post-C-section actually has a number of benefits and should be a priority for you and the staff caring for you. The longer we lay around, the higher our chances of developing blood clots, constipation, and pneumonia. Movement also stimulates the blood flow to the areas of the body that need to heal. The more blood being directed to the tissues that are disturbed during the cesarean surgery, the more oxygen and nutrients will arrive at the site, speeding the tissue repair.

Gentle movement daily will be an important part of the healing process, but that does not mean pushing a stroller for a walk in the neighborhood until you have been cleared for exercise. Besides potentially damaging the sutures internally, more rigorous exercise will shunt blood away from the abdomen to the working muscles, taking the blood flow away from the healing tissues and the digestive system, therefore slowing the healing process. Listen to your doctor and listen to your body. Ask for help when getting up, and for the first 24 hours, don't get up without a hand to hold on to if possible.

Postoperative Pain Management

Pain is not something you should simply accept as a part of the deal. Your approach to pain management should be strategic. Here is where being "in the know" will help you feel better much faster! As a general rule, you'll most likely be given narcotics through shots or a PCA (patient-controlled analgesia, which is a handheld trigger that releases a small amount of the drugs intravenously when pressed by the patient—controls are put in place to limit the dosage amount as well as the intervals at which the medication is released) for the first 12 to 24 hours postsurgery, after which it is likely that you will be prescribed pain medication in the form of a pill.

MOM to MOM: POSTSURGERY PAINKILLERS

After my first C-section, I thought I would try to take as little of the prescribed painkillers as possible—not a good move. For the first few days, allowing the pain medication to wear off completely before deciding to take another dose might not be the best idea. Good advice is to follow the dosing recommendations from your doctors and nurses. This will allow you to focus on bonding with your baby and allow you to be comfortable enough to sleep so the healing process can begin. It is very important to your health that you are comfortable enough to get up and walk around every few hours the day of and the day after your surgery to prevent blood clots and pneumonia. The painkillers will help make sure you can do that.

Remember, there are no medals awarded for going without some form of medication. I have never been one to take medicine unnecessarily, and I don't promote being overmedicated at all. But I also realize that there is a time and place for everything, including medication. ~Mary Beth

The seven layers of the abdomen in which incisions are made all react differently to the surgery. Some swell more than others, some react differently to pain medication than others, and some heal faster or slower than others. Knowing this will help you take the right approach, use the right type of medication, and move about with as little discomfort as possible.

The first thing you need to determine about your postoperation pain is what type of pain you are having. It is completely normal to feel many different pain sensations (such as pulling, tugging, burning, aching, and, less often, sharp pain)—after all, seven layers of tissue were disturbed to deliver the baby, and your body is trying to reverse the changes that pregnancy brought. It is a tremendous amount of work!

One more piece of advice when it comes to pain management and pain medication: Keep a journal! For the first few days after Mazie's birth, I didn't know whether I was coming or going, or if it was day or night. And had I not written down my medication, the dose and the time at which I took it last, I would not have had a clue. I would have underestimated the time in an effort to not overmedicate myself, which would have left me suffering between doses for no reason. Writing down (or having your partner or spouse write down) your medication will help you keep the appropriate schedule, which will aid in your staying comfortable. Not only is this great for you, but it is also a great procedure to have in place long before your baby needs to take medication for the first time!

Skin Deep

The skin is the first layer to be damaged and the last to heal. The healing process will take place from the inside out, systematically re-knitting each and every layer. At your post–C-section checkup, your doctor will take a good look at the incision to make sure the healing process has begun. This lets the doctor know that the layers below are further along in the healing process. Although the incision will not be pretty and you will have noticeable discomfort, there is no need to worry unless the incision begins to bleed, ooze, smell bad, or open.

What Will the Scar Look Like and Feel Like?

The incision will be red, itchy, and most likely puffy—but avoid scratching it! You will no doubt leave the hospital with surgical tape over the entire incision or parts of it. After a few days, the tape will easily peel away. Forcing it off will feel like a bad bikini wax; so don't bother. You might as well let it loosen on its own and then remove it without adding insult to injury.

> ### MOM TO MOM: TAKE THE PAIN MEDS
> If I were to give other C-section moms one piece of advice it would be to take the pain meds! I have never needed narcotics before my labor and was very hesitant to take them because I tend to have a bad reaction. I started with the smallest dose they would let me take, but by eight hours later was begging for the strongest dose. I would tell women not to worry about taking them because you only need them a short time. I was done with them a week after I had the baby.
> ~Tiffany

The incision and stitches in the skin will most likely leave you with a stinging or pulling sensation. Oftentimes a burning feeling will occur as well, like an abrasion or scrape. This burning sensation will fade over the next few days and will be replaced by an itching sensation. This itching sensation is a sign of growth—that the tissues are re-knitting themselves and the healing process is well under way.

Relief for a Painful or Swollen Scar

Applying ice packs to the scar not only alleviates pain, but also shrinks the swelling, which may reduce the tugging sensation. Be sure to put a layer of fabric (a washcloth, for example) between the pack and your scar, helping to keep the incision dry and the skin from suffering further irritation from an ice burn. Taking your prescribed pain medication for the first few days will also greatly reduce the discomfort felt at the skin.

After the pain medication is completely out of your system, you will most likely experience a sensation of numbness and/or tingling around the scar. This numbness will stay with you for the better part of six to nine months. The sensations stem from the fact that nerves were cut during the surgery and they need time to regenerate. The numbness and tingling will fade as the nerves heal.

The Uterus

Uterine cramping will occur in the weeks after childbirth in the effort of returning the uterus to its normal size. Moms who are breast-feeding may find that they experience uterine cramping in the midst of feeding, as the nipple stimulation increases the rate at which the uterus returns to its normal size. The hormone oxytocin, which stimulates milk flow, also makes the uterus contract.

Relief for Pain in the Uterus

Both the uterine cramping and pain caused from the incision in the uterus are best treated with consistent, daily use of ibuprofen (such as Advil or Motrin). These types of medication alleviate the pain and lessen the swelling at the site of the incision on the uterine wall. If you are inconsistent and take the ibuprofen every other day, you run the risk of minimizing inflammation one day and then allowing it to come back the next. This cycle of pain, relief, and then more pain may continue until the healing process is complete. Inflammation causes pain and minimizing pain means being consistent in your approach. Ask your physician for recommendations, as he or she knows you and your body best.

Gas Pain, Bloating, and the Digestive System

Many moms, including me, experience sharp pains in the chest and shoulders; others might notice the pain and bloating in the abdomen. The discomfort may begin during surgery and can potentially last for days afterward. This particular type of pain is caused by air having entered the abdominal cavity. This pain will subside as the air leaves the cavity. It is not dangerous and is treated best by gentle movements and a healthy fibrous diet and proper fluid intake. If intestinal gas pain does not subside, your nurse or doctor might recommend an over-the-counter medication containing Simethicone to help you begin to expel the gas and feel some relief.

MOM to MOM: DEALING WITH GAS

I guess the most surprising part of the experience was the pain I was in due to all the abdominal gas. The nurses kept telling me not to be shy about passing it, but I had trouble coordinating the muscles to get it out. That part was not fun. I am a physical therapist, so the actual surgery was not that bad for me; I'm used to all the medical stuff. I am also a big fan of A Baby Story on TLC so I had watched lots of C-sections on that show and knew the basics.

I wish I would have known that I had to stay in bed for 12 hours after the surgery. I didn't really feel like getting up anyway and it was funny watching my husband change all the gross diapers, but I just didn't realize I would have to stay in bed. I would encourage women to walk the hallways as soon as they'll let you. It helped me pass the gas and have my first bowel movement, which was also not an easy task. ~Anita

Relief for Digestive Disturbances

The peritoneum is a very sensitive layer of soft tissue, and two layers of this are disturbed during surgery. Abdominal discomfort due to bloating and an irritable bowel is not uncommon after surgery. The digestive system slows down considerably during surgery and recovery, and your bowels may not be functioning normally for many days, weeks, or even a month after the cesarean. Although an oxycodone with acetaminophen (such as Percocet) may help to ease other discomforts, it can often aggravate the digestive system further, increasing constipation. These ideas may help:

- Take an antacid (Mylanta or Maalox, for example).
- Reestablish a healthy digestive tract with yogurts such as Dannon's Activia. Containing Bifidus Regularis, this type of product may help normalcy return to your system much faster than just allowing nature to run its course.
- Engage in gentle movements. Changing positions frequently when in bed or on the couch as well as short walks around the house will help to alleviate both gas pains and intestinal malfunctions. Since you will not be released until after your first bowel movement, shorts walks should be on your to-do list.
- Stay on top of your fluid intake; this will help your digestive system return to normal. Dehydration can increase constipation and the discomfort associated with it.

Connective Tissues

Another layer of tissue that will cause you to experience discomfort is the fascia, the connective tissue that groups like muscle fibers together so that they can contract as one unit. The fascia of the abdomen is cut to allow the rectus abdominis halves to be moved aside. After the surgery, this tissue will swell, causing you to feel pressure in the abdomen, especially near your incision. You may notice a dull and consistent, somewhat vague sensation of pain from the fascia. Again, ibuprofen will help reduce the swelling and ease the pulling sensation.

Be Patient

The fascia does not have the blood flow that many other tissues do, and therefore it will most likely take the longest to heal. It is very important to allow for this layer to heal properly. Returning to exercise too soon, improperly exercising the abdominal muscles, lifting heavy items before the fascia is healed, and even slamming on the brakes in your vehicle (which is one of the reasons to heed your doctor's advice and not drive for a few weeks!) could all lead to the rectus abdominis muscle poking through the incision in the fascia, causing a hernia. The last place a C-section mom wants to be just weeks after surgery is back on the operating table. Take your time—and your doctor's advice—and allow for proper healing of each and every layer! For more information on proper exercise during the recovery period, read Chapter 3.

Your Transversus Abdominis

To help ease pain of sudden movements and occurrences such as coughing and sneezing, keep a pillow nearby and place it firmly against your abdomen when these actions occur. Simple bodily functions such as coughing and sneezing are reliant on the deepest muscle of the abdomen called the transversus abdominis. This muscle is also the one that is stretched out the most during pregnancy. Besides aiding in these functions, the transversus abdominis is one of your body's main stability muscles. Being overstretched from pregnancy, this muscle is not able to properly support your abdominal wall, leaving you at risk for overusing and injuring your back—yet another other reason to take it easy in the first few weeks postsurgery.

Scar Tissue

Keep in mind that any time injury occurs to tissues in the body, scar tissue is formed to help fill the gap that the damaged tissue left behind. All the layers of tissue in the abdomen are meant to float independently of each other. As scar tissue forms, it may not "lie down" properly. In other words, it may be thicker or bumpier than the original tissue it is replacing. This can cause two or more layers of the abdomen to adhere to each other, resulting in friction and a tugging sensation. Massage and myofascial release techniques (gentle, sustained pressure applied to fascia by pressing on the skin above the affected area) can help alleviate this condition. Trauma, inflammation, and surgery can create restrictions on the fascia that decrease movement, range of motion, and the ability to maintain proper posture. Cross friction, a form of medical massage, can also promote healing in that it works to break down scar tissues that may be preventing proper healing as well as encouraging the proper formation of scar tissues. Seek out an expert massage therapist or physical therapist who has experience in C-section recovery.

The Best Way to Heal: Sleep!

I know you are anxious to get home and start your new life as a mom, but if I could do it all over again, I would stay in the hospital as long as I was allowed! With an entire staff of nurses by your side, and one or two specifically assigned to you, this might be as much sleep as you get for the next 18 or so years. I kept both my babies in my hospital room with me the first night, feeling like I needed them close by to let the bonding kick in full force. By the second night, I realized that unless I slept, my surgery recovery was going to take longer than I wanted it to. So off to the nursery my babies went. They were lovingly cared for in the nursery (those nurses are so devoted!), and I was able to rest and be an even more doting and loving mom the next morning! It is vital that within the first day of motherhood you begin to grasp "mom guilt." Your heartstrings will be tugged 10,000 times a day (or more) for the rest of your life. You will be exhausted, unhappy, and lost if you give way to mom guilt each time and always choose your children first. Yes, they do come first—you are responsible for them—but they have to come after your health. If you are not well, they can't be either (at least not for the first few years, anyway). So take a deep breath and banish a little mom guilt every day, doing one thing for yourself that improves you—and sleep improves everything about you. One hundred percent of moms I surveyed wished they had stayed in the hospital as long as they could have. Most went home one day early, but all could have used another day before the rest of their lives began. There is no such thing as a perfect mom: Your friends aren't perfect, your mom's not perfect, and you won't be. You will try hard, as hard as you can, but always remember that you are as far from perfect as you can be when you are sleep-deprived.

The fact is, most of the body's healing process takes place at night while we sleep. Since many new moms are only capturing a few hours of shuteye at a time, recovery can be challenging to say the least. And even though you want the world to see just how beautiful your new baby is, the more visitors you have, the fewer minutes of rest you are getting. Space those visits out over a few weeks instead of during those first few days, and your body will thank you.

HOMEWARD BOUND

Be Prepared for a Rollercoaster of Emotions

Excitement and elation over the birth of your baby may have you flying high as you leave the hospital and head home three to four days after your C-section delivery. But you may also encounter fears and insecurities too. I remember when my husband and I placed Mazie in her crib (and watching her sleep for about 30 minutes), then headed for the couch to relax. Suddenly I began to cry. Eric asked me what was wrong, and I said "She's going to go to college some day. She's going to leave us." Eric laughed and commented that we had 18 years to go before that day came. Over the next few weeks I experienced many moments of happiness, sadness, success, failure, self-assuredness, and fear, as many new moms do. There were many highs and lows, physically and emotionally. While hormone fluctuations are difficult to manage, a little planning for the first week or two at home will help to manage the physical discomforts and get you back on your feet after surgery.

Symptoms to Watch For

Keep in mind that your recovery is a process, and it can take a month or two before you are fully healed. Most of the women that

I surveyed about their C-section experience rated the first week at home more challenging than the first 24 hours postsurgery. It's vital to have a plan and a good support system in place. In addition, it's important to know how to judge the progress of your healing so you can engage in the proper amount of activity, per your doctor's orders.

First things first: Recognize the signs that something isn't right. If the following symptoms occur, call your doctor!

- Low-grade fever lasting more than 24 hours.
- Fever of 101 degrees or more.
- Persistent pain. Discomfort is one thing; flat-out pain that does not diminish is another, and that is not acceptable! Do not think that you are being overdramatic or a wimp: Call your doctor.
- Drainage at the incision. While some may be normal, blood or pus means a visit to your doctor. Call, let your doctor know what you see, and make a visit to his or her office.
- Difficulty breathing. This may be a result of the surgery. If you are unable to take a deep breath, let your healthcare providers know.

Allow Others to Help, and Take It Easy

You are not the only one thrilled about your little baby. Friends and family not only can't wait to meet the little one, but they also truly want to lend a hand. *Let them!* Laundry, cleaning, cooking, and other household chores can potentially rob you of your energy to heal. Place your recovery at the top of your daily to-do list, and start dishing out the rest of the work.

Keep your hospital discharge papers handy to remind yourself to limit your activity. Here are some typical recommendations.

- **Avoid the stairs**, and basically live on one floor of your home. Only go up and down the steps one time per day. Living on one floor does require a little forethought so that you have what you need (a few diaper-changing stations are a must!).

- **Keep the baby close to you at night** so that you can get as much rest as possible (rather than spending time going back and forth to where the baby is to feed or comfort her).

- **Lift nothing heavier than your baby!** Banish the thought of carrying groceries, laundry, and even the baby in the car seat! A gallon of milk typically weighs 8 pounds; this is the heaviest (besides your baby) that you should be lifting.

- **Do not drive until your doctor tells you it is okay.** It is illegal to drive under the influence of many pain medications, and your reflexes may be slowed since the surgery, preventing you from reacting in time to avoid an accident. Suddenly slamming on the brakes might even cause internal damage or disrupt the healing process.

- **Avoid intercourse for six weeks.** Although you might emotionally be ready to reconnect with your partner, your body simply isn't.

- **Make sure you're drinking water throughout the day.** Sixty-four ounces is the bare minimum that you should be taking in. Dehydration will slow your healing process and leave you excessively fatigued. Add a slice of lemon, lime, or orange to your water. The potassium found in the fruit will help your body absorb the water and put it to good use.

- **Nap as often as you can**, and remind yourself that a catnap will be much better for you and your baby than another cup of coffee or sugary snack that will have you crashing down in no time. Although many new moms feel a sense of isolation during the first few months of motherhood (and who wouldn't, being stuck at home, unable to drive and recovering from surgery), your tissues heal faster at rest.

- **Limit the number of visitors you have daily.** Brenda Minica, a doula in San Antonio, Texas, advises her patients to stay in their pajamas. What a great idea! It reminds people that you are still healing. If your friends stop by for a while, they will no doubt make a comment such as, "We should go, and let you get some rest." You will no doubt say something like, "Oh, I'm fine," but you should really say, "Actually, I am pretty tired and do think a nap would help."

- **Journal.** The first weeks will fly by and will be but a brief memory, unless you capture them by writing or typing your experiences. Capturing both the good memories and the bad is important. Writing is a great way to let out the feelings that you may be having about your C-section and your first few weeks as a mom. Like it or not, almost everything that happens to women happens to us physically and emotionally. Bottling it all up inside may lead to hours of therapy down the line. Writing a few words a day might help you avoid negative feelings and, more important, can help you realize if you are suffering from any degree of postpartum depression.

  Journaling is a great tool to use to recognize symptoms, feelings, and habits, all of which will affect your mothering skills and abilities. We often don't realize how we are feeling until we have written it down, day after day after day. If you find you are writing the same negative feelings or painful sensations, you might need to talk to your doctor about them. Do not rely on your memory at this stage of the game! List the questions you have for your doctor at your first postoperation checkup and take it with you. Write down the doctor's response to them on the sheet so that you have something other than memory to fall back on.

- **Move daily!** Second-time mom, first-time C-section mom Natalie recalls this time to be a confusing one for her. She was told to limit activities and rest, yet move. Who wouldn't find that confusing? So what exactly should you make of these often conflicting statements?

Moving daily does not mean exercise! It means a simple walk to the mailbox or to the neighbor's house (assuming your neighbor lives less than a five-minute walk away) to show off your new baby (who is being pushed in a stroller by someone else!). Keep in mind the movement will speed the return of properly functioning bowels and intestines as well as potentially reduce gas pain and abdominal bloating that can linger for weeks postdelivery. Until you are cleared for exercise, make sure these walks are slow and that you are not carrying anything! In fact, for the first weeks at home you should keep your activity down to just moving around the house for a few minutes at a time.

MOM to MOM: MIDNIGHT SNACKS!

In those first few days home, I developed a habit that I now know aided greatly in my energy level, my ability to breastfeed, and my recovery. Each time I awoke for a middle-of-the-night feeding, I first made a trip to the bathroom, and then I went to the kitchen (only another 10 steps away) and grabbed a glass of water and a handful of graham crackers or Swedish fish (my weakness!). I had read that breastfeeding meant I was burning an additional 500 or so calories per day, and although I wanted to lose the baby weight, I also didn't want to feel horrible in doing so. My doctor and I also felt that this was not the time for a very low-calorie diet, which could not only slow the healing process but also affect my ability to produce breastmilk. Plus, every new mom deserves a little treat! There's no doubt in my mind that the additional fluid intake and the few extra calories prevented excess fatigue and grumpiness. ~Mary Beth

Daily Strategies for Healing

Before you begin any light exercising, remember that our bodies are highly adaptable, and they do not mind change when it takes place over a period of time. Our bodies do not like sudden change, however. Could you imagine if all the changes that occurred to your body during pregnancy took place overnight? How stressful would that be, not to mention horribly uncomfortable?

Yet one day, you are at full term in your pregnancy, and within hours, you're not pregnant! This is an enormous amount of change for one day, and as much as you can't wait to be your old self again, your body just isn't ready. It needs to take baby steps, regaining its abilities and its shape one day at a time. Don't rush the healing, and don't rush the return to fitness. Your body will appreciate your patient approach, and in the end, it will reward you by being there when you need it, and responding the way you want it to!

THE FIRST STEP: STRETCHING

A Week-by-Week Guide

Following are simple exercises to do once you come home from the hospital. Be sure to check with your doctor before beginning.

SURGERY RECOVERY WORKOUT			
	Stretches	Cardio	Core
Week 1: Perform all 1× per day	Toe Raises, Calf Stretches, Upper Back Stretch, Chest Stretch, Shoulder Stretch, Hamstring Stretch, Hip Flexor Stretch, Lower Back Stretch, Thigh Stretch, Tricep Stretch, Hip Stretch, Oblique Stretch	Walk for 3–5 minutes at the top of every hour.	Pelvic Tilts, Abdominal Compression, Kegels, One-Foot Balancing
Week 2: Perform all 2× per day	Toe Raises, Calf Stretches, Upper Back Stretch, Chest Stretch, Shoulder Stretch, Hamstring Stretch, Hip Flexor Stretch, Lower Back Stretch, Thigh Stretch, Tricep Stretch, Hip Stretch, Oblique Stretch	Walk for 3–5 minutes at the top of every hour. If energy allows, walk slowly and casually for 15 minutes 4 times over the week.	Pelvic Tilts, Abdominal Compression, Kegels, One-Foot Balancing
Week 3 until cleared for exercise: Perform all 2× per day	Toe Raises, Calf Stretches, Upper Back Stretch, Chest Stretch, Shoulder Stretch, Hamstring Stretch, Hip Flexor Stretch, Lower Back Stretch, Thigh Stretch, Tricep Stretch, Hip Stretch, Oblique Stretch	Walk for 3–5 minutes at the top of every hour. If energy allows, walk slowly and casually for 15 minutes 4 times over the week.	Pelvic Tilts, Abdominal Compression, Kegels, One-Foot Balancing, Pelvic Tilts with Bridge, Abdominal Compression with Leg Lift, Compression with Ball Squeeze, Leg Lifts

Week One

Strategy for week one is to increase the blood flow to the healing tissues while reminding our postural muscles of their jobs. Here are some exercises and stretches that will help facilitate this process.

WALKING

At the top of each waking hour, get up and walk around the house for 3 to 5 minutes to help promote healing, remove toxins, minimize constipation, and minimize the risk of blood clots. Set an alarm on your cell phone or use a kitchen timer as a reminder that it is time to move.

ONE-FOOT BALANCING

After moving about for a few minutes, practice balancing on one foot. Hold on to a countertop or the back of a chair, and simply lift one foot up off the ground and rest the foot against the inside of your opposite foot. After holding for 15 seconds, switch legs and repeat. Your center of gravity changed during pregnancy, and your body will need to readjust to the change in weight and weight distribution after delivery during the next few weeks.

TOE RAISES

While holding on to the counter or chair, lift up onto your toes and hold for 10 to 20 seconds before releasing. Perform 3 to 5 toe raises every other day.

CALF STRETCHES

Always follow the toe raises with a calf stretch. That way, in case you do not make it through the stretches listed below, at least you will have completed this one, which can prevent lower leg cramping, a common pre- and postnatal ailment. Using a wall, lift the toes of your right foot up off the ground, and rest them on the wall; keep your heel on the floor. Lean forward into the wall slightly. You should feel a stretch in the lower half of your leg. Hold for 10 to 20 seconds and release, then switch legs.

PELVIC TILTS

Pelvic tilts are a great way to begin addressing the muscular weakness and postural changes that occur during pregnancy, and they can be done in bed before you get up in the morning. Your lower back has a natural curvature to it; a pelvic tilt will reduce that curve. Imagine that your pelvis is a bucket of water. While you are in this starting position, the water will not "spill" out of the bucket. Tip the top of the bucket back, flattening your back into the bed or the floor, letting the water spill out of the back of the bucket. As you tilt back, gently draw your navel to your spine. Then release to the beginning position and repeat 5 to 8 times. Pelvic tilts can be done daily unless they are accompanied by pain or you notice an increase in vaginal bright red blood flow.

ABDOMINAL COMPRESSION

Abdominal compression is a good move to try if you are relatively pain-free. Again, you can perform these in bed each morning, prior to getting up. While on your back, bend your knees and bring your feet underneath them, flat on the bed. Draw your shoulders down toward the bed and keep your chin lifted out of your chest. Inhale through your nose, and as you exhale through your mouth, draw your navel back toward your spine, slowly and gently. Do not flatten your lower back into the bed as you perform this compression. Instead keep the natural arch. Visualize a grape under your lower back, and as you exhale, try not to crush the grape. You can also try to slide one of your hands under your lower back to see if you are indeed keeping the natural arch in your back. However do not lift your ribcage to do so. Do not worry if you cannot slide your hand under your back due to stretched-out tissues and the extra padding that you carried to maintain a healthy pregnancy and to prepare for becoming a food source. Within a few weeks to a month, you will be able to slide your hand right under your back!

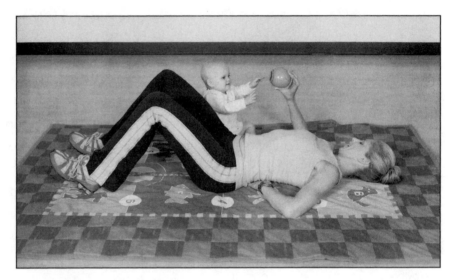

▲ ABDOMINAL COMPRESSION

Perform this compression of the abdomen 5 to 8 times twice a day to begin stabilizing your torso and alleviating overuse of the lower back. Try to make your inhales and exhales match in duration—breathing in and out for a count of 5 to ensure slow and controlled movements. Now is a great time to learn how to come to the realization that you may never have a moment to yourself for the next three years. That is why moms are great at multitasking. It is simple to perform this and other moves with your baby by your side. Due to abdominal sensitivity in the first few weeks I would not suggest doing these moves with your baby lying on your chest, but they can certainly lie by your side while you take care of you! Grab a rattle or their favorite stuffed animal and entertain them while you perform this and other moves.

KEGELS

You can start Kegels in the first week you are home from the hospital. This great description of Kegels exercises (it can be hard to tell if you are doing them properly!) comes from WEBMD.com:

- "First, as you are sitting or lying down, try to contract the muscles you would use to stop urinating. You should feel your pelvic muscles squeezing your urethra and anus. If your stomach or buttocks muscles tighten, you are not exercising the right muscles.
- "When you've found the right way to contract the pelvic muscles, squeeze for 3 seconds and then relax for 3 seconds.
- "Repeat this exercise 10 to 15 times per session. Try to do this at least 3 times a day. Kegel exercises are only effective when done regularly. The more you exercise, the more likely it is that the exercises will help."

Lack of movement can lead to tight muscles; while your body is warm from the above gentle movements, gentle stretching is a must to alleviate poor pregnancy posture.

Stretches for Week 1

Perform the first three exercises below seated in a comfortable chair, or while kneeling on the floor. Either way is just fine. If getting up and out of bed by yourself is difficult in these first few weeks, then perform these in a chair until your mobility increases. If using a chair, sit upright, and do not lean back against the back of the chair. Feel free to place a pillow behind your lower back for support, but try not to rest your shoulders on the chair back.

UPPER BACK STRETCH

Interlock your fingertips, and push your palms out away from you (Figure 1). Round out your upper back, and drop your chin into your chest (Figure 2). Think about creating space between your shoulder blades. Hold for 5 deep breaths and release, returning to the starting position.

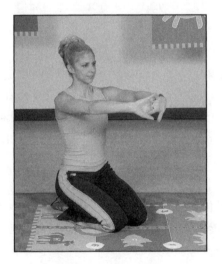

▲ UPPER BACK STRETCH,
FIGURE 1

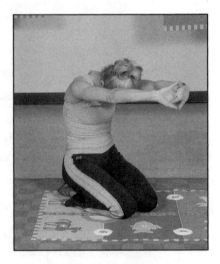

▲ UPPER BACK STRETCH,
FIGURE 2

CHEST STRETCH

With your fingers still interlocked, press your palms up toward the ceiling, bringing your arms alongside your ears. Take 5 deep breaths as you elongate your torso and then bring your interlocked fingers down to the base of your neck (Figure 1). Press your elbows back, and let the weight of your head be felt in your hands (Figure 2). Breathe deeply 5 times before releasing your hands to your sides.

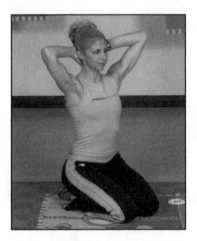
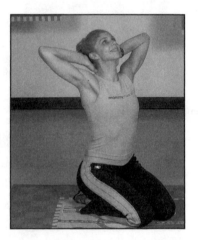

▲ CHEST STRETCH, FIGURE 1   ▲   CHEST STRETCH, FIGURE 2

SHOULDER STRETCH

Bring your interlocked hands behind your lower back, roll your shoulders down and back, gently lifting your hands up off the lower back. Hold for 5 deep inhales and exhales. If flexibility does not allow you to interlock your hands, feel free to hold each elbow in the palm of the opposite hand and hold for 5 deep inhales and exhales.

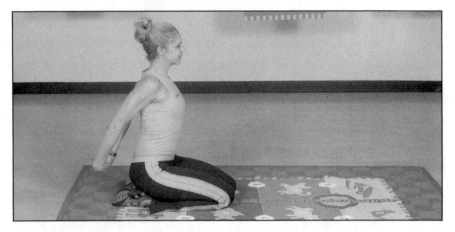

▲ SHOULDER STRETCH

TRICEPS STRETCH

Sit on the floor with your legs tucked underneath you. Stretch your right arm up to the ceiling (Figure 1), then bend at the elbow and reach your right fingertips toward the middle of your upper back. Pull back gently on your right elbow with your left hand (Figure 2). Hold for 20 seconds and then release, repeating on the other side.

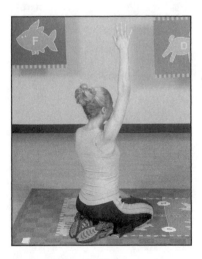

▲ TRICEPS STRETCH, FIGURE 1

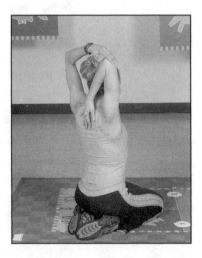

▲ TRICEPS STRETCH, FIGURE 2

HAMSTRING STRETCH

In a seated position on the floor, begin by flexing your feet (Figure 1). Pull your toes back toward your body, and slowly lean forward, keeping your chin lifted and your knees slightly bent. Keep your feet properly aligned (toes facing straight forward and hips squared). Reach your hands out for your lower legs and grab hold of them (Figure 2). Hold for 20 seconds and then slowly release.

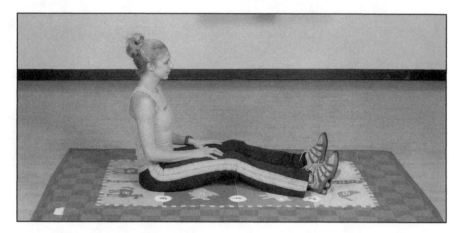

▲ HAMSTRING STRETCH, FIGURE 1

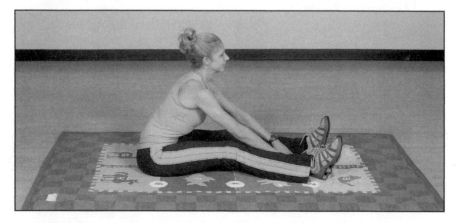

▲ HAMSTRING STRETCH, FIGURE 2

HIP STRETCH

Cross your right ankle over your left knee as shown. Gently press down on your right knee, feeling a stretch in the outer hip on the right side. Hold for 20 seconds, release, and switch sides. Lean forward slightly to increase the stretch.

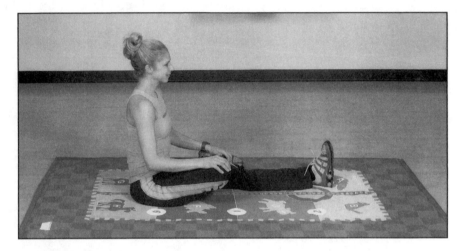

▲ HIP STRETCH

HIP FLEXOR STRETCH

Begin in a kneeling position, and take your right foot out in front of you. Lean forward, bringing the right knee out over the right toes. You should feel a slight stretch down the front of the hip. To increase the stretch, move your shoulders back over your hips and extend your left arm up and over the midline of your body. Hold for 20 seconds then release and switch sides. A slight tugging around your scar is normal; pain is not. If this stretch causes pain, ease out of it and try it again in 5 to 7 days.

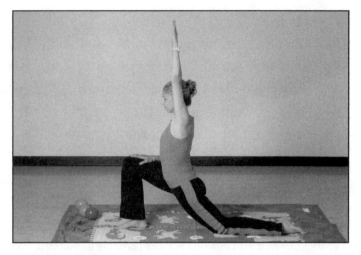

▲   HIP FLEXOR STRETCH

LOWER BACK STRETCH

Sitting or lying down for long periods of time causes the back to tighten up. Perform this stretch a few times a day to keep your low back loose. Come to a kneeling position on the floor, sit down on the back of your feet, and round your spine, bringing your forehead toward the floor. Place your hands by your feet and let the weight of your body sink into the floor. Hold this stretch for 5 deep breaths.

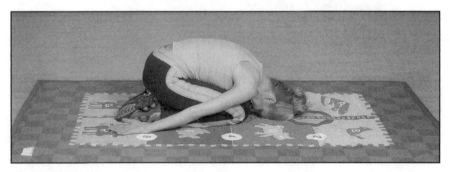

▲ LOWER BACK STRETCH

THIGH STRETCH

I found that doing this stretch while lying on my side in bed was the easiest way to move in and out of the stretch in the first two weeks after surgery. It can also be done standing if flexibility allows. While lying on your right side, have your partner or friend place a pillow behind your upper back to prevent you from rolling onto your back. Lift your left leg up just a few inches, bend at the knee, and bring your heel back toward your rear end. Hold on to your left foot with your left hand. You should feel a stretch down the front of your left leg. Hold for 20 seconds and then release. Switch to the other side, using pillows to prevent rolling over, and repeat the stretch.

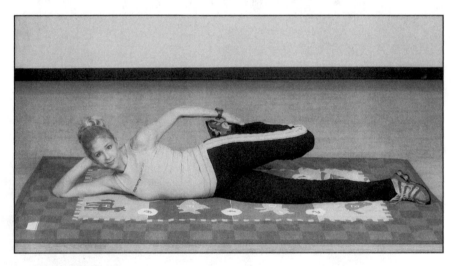

▲ THIGH STRETCH

OBLIQUE STRETCH

Sit on the floor in a cross-legged position. Place your left hand on right knee and extend your right hand over your head, dropping your left shoulder closer to the floor. Hold for 20 seconds and release, repeating on the other side. When your baby is able to sit up on his own, place him in front of you and use the arm crossing in front of the body to support him.

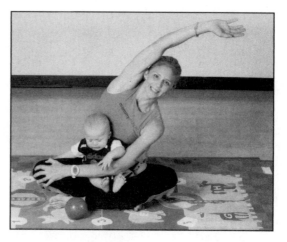

▲   OBLIQUE STRETCH

Week Two

All of the stretches and abdominal compressions that you performed in week one should be carried over and performed in week two. Now, however, perform them twice a day to decrease your recovery time.

As long as you have enough energy, walk 4 to 5 times a week for 15 to 20 minutes. Start with 15 minutes of gentle walking (not breaking a sweat). Try this the first few times. If your energy is good, and you are not experiencing any increase in bleeding or having any other warning signs discussed on page 32 or presented to you by a health professional, increase your duration to 20 minutes per walk. Remember, these are walks for healing and getting out of the house for fresh air, not walks for fat burning and getting the baby weight off!

Week Three until You Are Cleared for Exercise

It is important that you continue your routine from weeks one and two when it comes to stretching and walking until you are cleared for further exercise. Most C-section moms are cleared for exercise by the time they are six weeks postpartum. From week three until you are cleared for exercise, it is generally safe to add the following moves into your daily routine to begin gently increasing abdominal strength and pelvic stability as well as adding a new dimension to your pelvic floor strengthening moves.

- Pelvic tilts with bridge
- Abdominal compression with leg lift
- Compression with ball squeeze
- Leg lifts

Don't forget that all of these moves can be done with your bundle of joy right by your side. As a matter of fact, their bodies are learning to progress as well. At this stage they are beginning to recognize sounds and voices. As she is learning to focus, you may want to hold her favorite stuffed animal over her head and move it slowly from side to side, allowing the object to come in and out of her view. I loved doing this with Mazie and Miles and cheered when they began to turn their heads to follow the toy I was holding.

PELVIC TILTS WITH BRIDGE

Lying on your back on a comfortable surface, bend your knees, and place your feet on the floor, shoulder distance apart. Inhale, and as you exhale, perform an abdominal compression and lift your hips up off the ground, pushing them toward the ceiling. Perform 10 pelvic tilts in this bridge position. Think about the bucket of water as you scoop your pelvis under, trying to spill the water out the back side of the bucket, and then returning it to a neutral pelvic position.

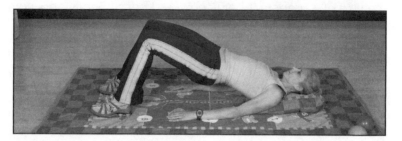

▲ PELVIC TILTS WITH BRIDGE

ABDOMINAL COMPRESSION WITH LEG LIFT

While on your back, bend your knees and bring your feet underneath them, flat on the floor, bed, or exercise mat. Draw your shoulders down, and keep your chin lifted. Inhale through your nose, and as you exhale through your mouth, draw your navel back toward your spine. Slowly and gently, lift your right foot off the bed or floor, bringing your right knee over your hip, and hold it here for 5 deep breaths. Keep your right shin parallel to the ceiling. Do not flatten your lower back into the bed as you perform this compression; instead, keep the natural arch. After completing 3 sets of 5, switch and complete 5 of them with your left leg.

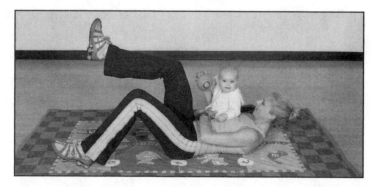

▲ ABDOMINAL COMPRESSION WITH LEG LIFT

COMPRESSION WITH BALL SQUEEZE

Following the compression exercises, place a small squeezable ball the size of a grapefruit between your knees. Gently apply pressure on the ball, bringing your knees closer together. Hold this isometric contraction (when the muscle contracts but does not shorten, therefore no movement takes place) of the inner thigh muscles for 10 seconds and slowly release. Repeat 3 times.

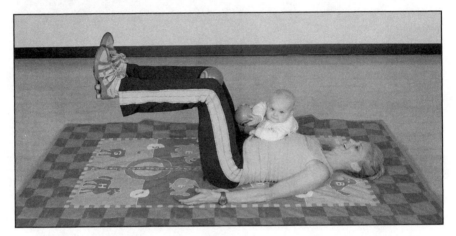

▲ COMPRESSION WITH BALL SQUEEZE

LEG LIFTS

This is a good one to do right after the Thigh Stretch on page 48. Before turning over to stretch the other leg, perform a few leg lifts. Inhale, and as you exhale, lift your top leg up about 3 inches and hold. Keep your leg straight, and do not allow for any rotation of the leg at the hip. Hold for 10 seconds and then lower the leg down to the resting position. Repeat 3 times on each leg.

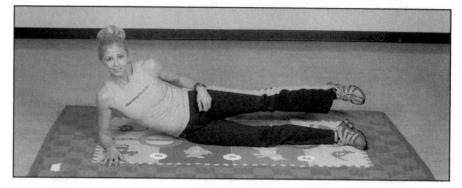

▲ LEG LIFT

Listen to Your Body!

If you experience abdominal or pelvic pain, lightheadedness, dizziness, or nausea while performing these moves at any point, stop immediately. If symptoms persist, call your doctor. Review the postsurgery warning signs and symptoms from your doctor, and heed his or her advice. Time heals all wounds, including those from C-section deliveries. You too will heal, and you too will reclaim your body and have the ability to like it better than before pregnancy, if you progress slowly and listen to your body. Drink lots of fluids and rest. Your body, mind, and spirit are not just in a recovery and healing phase, but they are also working hard to acclimate to all of the new demands on your life, your time, and your energy. It might take a few weeks to find your rhythm for this stage of life, but it will come.

WHY YOU NEED TO EXERCISE

Facing a Choice

As a new mom (whether the baby is your first, second, third, or fourth), you are going to face quite a challenge in finding time, energy, and the desire for exercise. With each addition to the family, a mom's life seems to become less and less her own. We do not seem to mind the loss of our own lives at the end of each day when we know in our hearts and in our minds that we have taken proper care of our families and given them our best. It is this kind of selfless behavior that helps to shape our children, and in some way, helps to shape our country, since our children are its future! Losing part of ourselves in our children and their lives is a part of the role we play.

Losing yourself *completely*—putting your health and well-being on the shelf—is not, or should not be, part of the role. What you, as a mom, must understand is that your body and your life are still yours. You determine the outcome for both. If you choose to lose yourself completely in your family, you will. You can raise your kids to be great young people, and then the day they head off to college, you'll have *no* idea who you are or what to do. You can also choose not to take care of your body—it's easy to blame it on time, money, energy, and so on. But if you let your health fall by the wayside, you increase your risk of obesity, along with many other diseases that have the potential to shorten your life span, giving you fewer minutes on this Earth with the precious beings that you helped to bring into it. Personally, I want as many happy memories with my children as possible. Therefore, I choose to exercise and do my best to eat right.

You can also choose to feel less than approving of your new-mom body. The same body that was graced with the ability to produce life can become your best friend or your worst enemy during motherhood, and the choice is yours. Exercise is not an option. It is a must for everyone, but especially so for moms. Outside of the physical benefits, the emotional gains are too great to deny yourself a regular exercise program. It is my firm belief that a mom who has a strong, confident body will instill strength, confidence, and good self-esteem in her children.

Accepting Your Postpregnancy Size

I will never forget leaving the hospital with Mazie. She was so tiny and I was so not! After two full days of having fluid pumped into my body intravenously, I felt like a blowfish. I was retaining so much fluid that, three days after giving birth via C-section, I left the hospital a half pound lighter than I went in. A half of a pound! I had women telling me for nine months that I would lose 20 of the 50 pounds I had gained before even leaving the hospital! I was so sure that my body would bounce back quickly that I brought a medium-sized sweatsuit to the hospital to wear home. Dejected, I wore maternity pants home and had to put on one of my husband's dress shirts because the maternity top I wore there was too small. At that time I did not know enough about the body to understand this process, and without the knowledge, I spent weeks worrying that perhaps I wouldn't lose the baby weight.

I was especially worried because I had really struggled with my weight gain (during both pregnancies). Again, the voice of others saying "You're so active, you probably won't gain more than 25 pounds" rang in my head. I wish! Like many women, I gained just under 50 pounds with each of my children, and fear was building. I didn't want to be heavy again. I tried to reassure myself that I would lose every pound. "I am a fitness professional," I thought. "I help people lose weight for a living, I will lose the baby weight!" And I was right—*eventually*. But looking in the mirror for the first time after becoming a mom was not the most reassuring moment, and I began to wonder where my confidence and strength went. Had I let myself stay in this negative state, I may never have found the time, energy, or desire to exercise again. That's why it's important to acknowledge all the hard work your body has just gone through, and accept that it's okay if you're not even close to your prepregnancy size immediately. Stay focused on internal health and well-being and the reflection in the mirror will change.

Setting a Good Example

Overcoming the innate "mom-guilt" to take care of your body is vital to your own sanity and your ability to raise healthy, happy kids. Each and every one of us deserves to start off our day by walking into our closets and having everything fit the way we want it to. The way your clothes fit and the size of them plays a role in your self-esteem, like it or not. When your clothes fit right and you feel good about your body, you carry yourself with pride. When they don't fit or you begrudgingly move up a size, a little piece of your heart sinks, your brain registers the disappointment, and sometimes your spirit can't shake it. You might even think, "What happened to me? Where did I go and will I ever be back?"

Some days you probably don't even have the energy to realize how you feel about your body, and so you bury the thought and hope that someday you will look and feel like you used to. You might even think to yourself, "Well, at least my children look good!" If your spirit is dampened by the size of your clothes or the unfamiliarity of your own body, then you must take control of your life, find the time and energy to exercise, and realize that by taking better care of yourself, you can better care for your children.

If you are not strong and confident, how do you raise strong, confident children? If you do not spend time taking care of yourself, how do you teach your kids that they are important enough for a little time each day to honor their body and spirit? If you do not exercise and eat right, how can you possibly expect them to grow up with those habits?

Not only do you need to exercise, but you must also make exercise as regular of an activity as brushing your hair or teeth. Obesity is out of control in this country, and women during the child-bearing years are at a higher risk of obesity due to weight gained for pregnancy. And even though you may refer to this gain as "the baby weight," it can stay with you for the rest of your life if you let it. It is easy to let yourself believe that a few extra pounds from pregnancy are no big deal, but keeping 5 to 15 pounds from each pregnancy can add up to real health issues and increase the risk of diabetes, heart disease, and many forms of cancer.

Believe me, I know there are a thousand reasons why you don't want to exercise and hundreds of excuses presented each day to not exercise. Getting around these reasons and past the excuses can be tricky. For me, reminding myself of all the good that exercise does for my body and for my kids is what always gets me out the door. Once you know all the positive effects of exercise, you might be more inclined to participate daily. Following are some of the most compelling reasons to exercise.

MOM to MOM: I CHOSE A C-SECTION FOR MY TWINS

My C-section was planned and was my choice! I was having twins and I knew that the delivery could be tricky. I had so many other things to worry about that I didn't want this to be one of them. I became pregnant through IVF (in vitro fertilization) and had a rough pregnancy. I developed hypermesis gravarium (severe morning sickness) and needed an IV as well as a Zofran pump (a device that delivers antinausea medication) attached to my belly until I was 14 weeks along. To make matters worse, I also had hyperstimulated ovaries and my abdomen filled with so much fluid that at six weeks pregnant, I looked like I was six months along!

I was put on bed rest at 27 weeks because of preterm labor. Having developed the fear that I would deliver one baby vaginally then need a C-section for the second, I opted for the easiest choice. At 35.5 weeks, I delivered both girls via C-section easily one minute apart. Brooklyn weighed 4 pounds, 11 ounces and Marley weighed 3 pounds, 2 ounces. Due to her tiny size, Marley was in the NICU for a week before she was able to go home. I had no idea prior to their birth that if there are complications, like Marley's low birth-rate, and the baby(s) are in the NICU, that I wouldn't be able to get up and go see the baby until the next day. It broke my heart! I begged for my catheter to be removed so that I could get up and see Marley. The next day they removed it and I was up and down the hall in no time! I certainly had incentive to get up and get moving and I believe it played a big role in my speedy recovery. ~Katie

Stress Reduction

Every mom's life is stressful. I have yet to meet one who lives on Easy Street. Our days are filled with thousands of chores to do and hundreds of needs to fill, and only two hands, one heart, and one mind to complete them. We all carry and manage stress differently, but one common thread binds us: We will have happier moments every day if we learn to understand the physical assault that stress has on our bodies and how to reverse it. Not only will we be happier, but we will also be lighter!

The Biology of Stress

Everyone is born with the "fight" or "flight" reaction built in, and each time you encounter a stressful situation (recognized or not), your body reacts. The strategy for dealing with stress must first come in recognizing it, and then in managing it. Many situations can cause your internal bells and whistles to go off, such as a large dog barking at you while on a walk, performing the finger sweep on your baby who placed a small toy piece in his mouth the one second you had you back turned, or slamming on the brakes to avoid hitting a deer that wandered into your path. Those bells and whistles begin your body's chain reaction to stress. A gland near the base of your brain called the hypothalamus sends a signal to your adrenal glands to release a powerful combination of cortisol and adrenaline.

Whenever I think of adrenaline, the image of the Incredible Hulk comes to mind. Adrenaline can boost your strength and courage, enabling the fight-or-flight instinct by increasing your heart rate and quickening the pace at which your body delivers energy to each cell. For a mom, this means finding the speed to run into the street and pull a child out of the way of a car, or rushing to the changing table just in time to keep that baby who couldn't turn over yesterday from roll-ing off today! While adrenaline can help the body react quickly to a stressful encounter, allowing it to hang around for a few days after the trauma will do your body no good.

Your cortisol levels also increase in your system as you react to stress. An overproduction of cortisol as a result of too much stress can negatively affect many functions in the body. Your body is constantly reprioritizing itself to put the most important functions first. Most important to the body is brain function, for it controls all other func-tions in the body. Avoiding harm and removing yourself from stressors is also a high priority for the body and is part of your survival mecha-nism. Because there is only a certain amount of energy available for use at any given time, in the form of blood sugars (glucose), which system in the body gets the energy and for what purpose is what the brain is constantly reevaluating.

When faced with stress, the fight-or-flight instinct kicks into over-drive, cortisol elevates the amount of sugars in the blood stream, and your brain begins to use more of the blood sugars (glucose). Since brain function and the physical efforts needed to remove the stress are of top priority, glucose is diverted from other organs and tissues to the brain and the muscles. This diversion of glucose can suppress the immune system, digestive system, and the reproductive system. This is exactly why people are more likely to succumb to illness, encounter diges-tive irregularities, and possibly encounter difficulties conceiving when faced with repeated exposure to stress.

It is also important to note that the fight-or-flight reaction in your body sends messages to the part of your brain that deals with mood, fear, and motivation, which is why exposure to stress for short- or long-term periods can cause mood swings, lack of motivation, and increased sensitivity to everything you encounter. Heart disease, obesity, depression, memory loss, sleep deprivation, and digestive problems are the side effects of overexposure to stress. Repeated exposure to stress can also trigger food cravings, because any time your body uses blood sugars, they must be replaced. Repeated use of blood sugars in your reaction to stress causes a greater need for replenishment of them. If they are not replenished quickly enough, food cravings will set in and will not go away until the needed energy has been gained. Unfortunately, food cravings can and will get the better of you and often cause overeating of foods you shouldn't be eating in the first place. For a new mom wishing to lose the baby weight, these cravings can have the scale heading in the wrong direction.

Overcoming Stress

How we handle stress in our lives is based on both genetics and life experience. Whatever your reaction may be, it is important that you actively participate in reducing the effects of stress. Many articles have been written about reducing the stressors in our lives—and oh, how we wish we could! If you can, do it! Most of us, especially new moms, do not have that option. Those stressors are here to stay. This is where stress management becomes key.

Think of *moderate* cardiovascular exercise as active recovery from stress. Keeping your exercise moderate is vital to stress reduction. Overexertion during exercise increases levels of stress in the body and dumps more cortisol, which also signals the body to store fat instead of burn it—the opposite of what most of us want from exercise. During exercise, if you are huffing and puffing, become red in the face, feel a burning sensation, and begin to wonder how long you can make it, chances are you are working out too hard and you are increasing the stress levels. Make sure you can talk, you are capable of holding your pace for an extended period of time, and—even though it is an effort and you might be sweating—you aren't putting forth so much effort that you hate it or can't handle it for much longer. I often put a piece of gum in my mouth as I begin my cardio session; if I get to the point where I need to spit out the gum, I am working too hard. If I can blow a bubble, then I am not working hard enough!

MOM to MOM: A BABY'S CRY AFFECTS YOUR HEART RATE!

After the birth of my son Miles, I had an eye-opening experience to stress, its effects, and even how much something as simple as a baby's cry could affect a mom's body. I was getting ready to head out the door for an evening jog right after putting Miles to bed. My goal was to rid my body of the baby fat, and so I wore a heart rate monitor to make sure I was working out at the right effort, which would enable me to burn fat for fuel. I put Miles down in his crib and happened to notice that my heart rate was at 86. I tiptoed down the hall, and just as I got to the top of the stairs, he wailed! It was a huge, loud, angry cry! As I turned back toward his room, I noticed that my heart rate had jumped to 113. Wow—scientific proof that a baby's cry really does affect a mom's mind and body. This was one of the most valuable lessons I have ever learned. It made me realize just how often I am exposed to stress, how much my body reacts to stress, and how even a cry from my child causes my body to react. ~Mary Beth

When you understand the tremendous impact stress has on your body, you are probably more likely to work daily to counter each and every stressful event. Envision your body flushing the cortisol, reducing the adrenaline, and becoming balanced. Increase your fluid intake on stressful days, play music that soothes your mind and soul, curl up with a good book if only for a few minutes, call a neighbor or friend and ask them to come over so that you can relax by taking a real shower (not a new-mom get wet, soap up, rinse, and get out shower), or sip a cup of decaf tea, savoring the aroma before every sip. If you have these strategies readily available, when stresses enter your body (as they will, a thousand times a day), you can manage them. If you don't reduce it, you will be on edge, be crabby, be tired, and will have a short fuse, none of which will allow you to be the mother, wife, daughter, or friend that you intend to be.

Exercise Helps You Sleep Better

There are two things that each and every mom I know needs and wants—more sleep and more energy! Good news! Moderate exercise delivers on both fronts.

There is no doubt in my mind that motherhood begins at conception, and some time before delivery, moms realize that good sleep habits are no longer easy to come by and are perhaps a thing of the past. Developing a sleep strategy is vital to enjoying motherhood, having a productive workday, and having the energy to create great memories for you and your family. Sleep is one of those things that you probably didn't think a lot about, but motherhood changes everything, including sleep. As if your baby's eating and sleeping habits aren't enough to interrupt your sleep—or at least shorten the length of it—stress, depression, hormones, and anticipation can all make a good night's sleep seem out of reach. Although some moms need fewer hours of sleep than others, Mayo Clinic researchers have found that too little sleep leads to an inability to concentrate, decreased physical capabilities, and impaired memory, all of which make a mom's multitasking lifestyle a bigger drain on your energy levels.

The Science of Sleep

That's why a mom's sleep strategy should include exercise. Exercise has been shown to improve production of a powerful neurotransmitter called serotonin, which impacts a number of bodily functions, including sleep. In her report "Serotonin and Its Uses," Andrea Byrd, a medical researcher, writes, "The functions of serotonin are numerous and appear to involve control of appetite, sleep, memory and learning, temperature regulation, mood, behavior (including sexual and hallucinogenic behavior), cardiovascular function, muscle contraction, endocrine regulation, and depression." Your body needs sleep—when you are sleep-deprived and serotonin levels decrease, so does your ability to exercise and make smart food choices, thus diminishing the likelihood of weight loss. It is clear that the increased production of serotonin has a very positive effect on your body and in the end plays a very important role in weight loss and/or weight management.

Since exercise improves the body's production of serotonin, and serotonin helps control sleep, you're also sleeping better when you exercise, helping you to feel more rested in the morning. Restful sleep also lowers the risk of overeating because when you are fatigued, you are more likely to reach for foods laden with sugar or starch to give you a quick energy boost. The problem is this energy boost is followed by an enormous crash, from which you will probably need food or caffeine to recover. This merry-go-round of using calories and caffeine to sustain you for the day can lead to weight gain, mood swings, and more disruptive sleep patterns. That's why it's so important to understand the connection between sleep and weight.

There is another important tie-in for sleep and weight loss: Your body only builds lean muscle and repairs muscle (as well as other connective tissues that were disturbed during your C-section surgery) during non-REM sleep stages 3 and 4. Muscle burns, on average, five times as many calories a day as fat tissue, which means the more muscle you have, the more you can eat without gaining weight. The addition of lean muscle from strength training increases your ability to lose weight and keep it off. No worries, ladies—without an influx of supplements, some of which are illegal, the likelihood that a woman will bulk up from weight training is slim. Slim is actually the end result of weight training. Muscle is a far more compact and metabolically active tissue than fat, and for that reason, adding muscle is a must for sustained weight loss. Since your body cannot repair and build lean muscle without entering deeper stages of sleep, it is necessary to have a strategy for sleep when you are a mom.

How to Get More Sleep

Start planning out the ways that you can get a full night's sleep. Have your partner take turns with you for those nighttime feedings, or ask a friend or relative to come and stay with you one or two nights a week so that they can help with the baby in the middle of the night and you can wake up rested and repaired. Emotionally, this may be a challenge for new moms who want to breastfeed each and every time their baby needs nourishment. However, it will serve your body and your baby better both now and years down the line if you sleep now!

Reading this chapter is one thing; putting it into practice is yet another. But one thing is for certain: Life will not get any easier, and you will not like your body any better, if you don't work on sleep habits and stress management. I often hear my own mother's voice and the voices of other knowing moms who urged me to nap during the day when my babies were napping. Looking back, I wish I had. The dishes and the laundry will get done, you will finish that work project, and your friends and family who stop in to see you and the baby really don't care if your floor is spotless or not. The dishes will never be a matter of life or death, but lack of sleep and lack of exercise increase your risk of disease. They are a matter of life, they are a matter of more time with your family, and they are a matter of quality of life.

An empty sink has never made me feel as good or as energized as a 15-minute walk. Making all the beds in the house each day has never cleared my mind or improved my self-esteem like 20 minutes of weight training. And a perfectly kept bedroom will not build the muscle you need to sustain the weight loss like proper sleep will. Learn to rethink your new life as a mom. Your mental, physical, and emotional health must be at the top of your daily to-do list!

The Energy Equation

Though I do have some days when I need little convincing to exercise, I have many others when I have to mentally run through the list of all of the benefits of exercise before I can get myself moving. It is on those days that I remind myself of one of the biggest benefits of exercise—expending energy through exercise will give me more energy!

It's hard to believe, but it's true! Exercise can stimulate your system as much as caffeine, and it is often a better alternative, especially late in the afternoon or in the early evening when caffeine intake might delay your ability to fall asleep or stay asleep. Retrain your brain to recognize that exercise will give you a boost of energy. It is like having your very own jetpack. Revving up your body with a brisk walk or strength training session will have each system in your body operating at a higher, faster level. Regular exercise makes your body more efficient, meaning that even though you use energy during your exercise session, the increased functioning capacity of your body afterward causes you to use less energy for each and every other second of the day. This daily conservation of energy results in you having the energy to pursue your interests and hobbies after the kids are down for the night.

Physical efficiency can be hard to grasp. Here is an example of how it works. Movement requires the breakdown of energy for fuel, and that energy comes in the form of calories. The more fit you are, the fewer calories (energy) it takes to move you, and the more tissue your body consists of (the bigger you are), the more calories you need for movement. That's why whatever weight you keep on long-term after the baby might not bother your emotional or spiritual life, but it does have an effect on you physically. The extra weight causes you to expend more energy than necessary for movement. Losing weight is one of the easiest ways to gain energy!

Efficiency is the second way you can end the day with more energy and feel as if you can actually have a life outside of motherhood. Being physically efficient means that you use fewer calories for daily tasks and for exercise. For example, think about how many times you go up and down a flight of stairs a day. (Some days I am up and down the steps 15 times *before* leaving for work. Many times I have a child, laundry, or "load" in my arms.) For the sake of this example, let's assume you burn 5 calories going up the steps each time and you go up 15 times a day; this means that you have used 75 calories of energy. After performing cardiovascular exercise during which you are exerting the same amount of or a little more energy than going up the steps, your body will become more efficient, and perhaps you will lower your energy usage to 3 calories per flight (or

45 total calories), for a savings of 30 calories. I know that doesn't seem like much, but your newfound efficiency will be with you for each and every moment of each and every day. This can translate into at least 100 to 200 calories conserved during your waking hours, which is plenty of energy you can then use to make dinner instead of going through the drive thru, to take an evening walk, to make a phone call to a friend, to play a game of tag with the kids, or to challenge your partner to a game of chess.

As long as you are exercising properly and regularly, your body will continue to grow more efficient, sacrificing less fuel, and, as a result, you will become increasingly energetic.

How Exercise Promotes Healing

Moderate exercise can have an amazing effect on healing. The function of your heart and lungs improves and accelerates with exercise. This acceleration means that with each beat of your heart, more oxygen and nutrients are being delivered to each and every cell in your body and, as a result, the healing process quickens. Exercise provides many benefits to a person healing, including:

- Exercise helps increase blood flow to the area being used. The extra blood flow fills the area with cells that help heal the injury. It also increases the oxygen level in the area to promote healing, and increases circulation, which removes debris and injured cells.
- Exercise will alleviate stiffness in injured areas. Moving the affected muscles prevents scar adhesions from forming and resulting in a severely stiff joint.

- Using the muscles prevents muscle atrophy, which can occur when muscles lose their shape and strength after an injury. Exercising helps the muscles remain strong even while healing.

In the case of a new mom recovering from a cesarean delivery, rest is vital, and so is movement. The scar tissue that develops as a natural part of the healing process can form improperly, and cause two layers of tissue to connect instead of remaining separate. This connection can result in a tugging sensation when you move. When your nurse or doctor tells you it is time to move, it is—and it is for a variety of reasons, healing being a big one!

Although moderate exercise can improve the healing process, intense exercise can slow the process. When you exercise at 85 percent or more of your maximum capacity (discussed in Chapter 9), blood and nutrients can be shunted away from healing tissues and directed toward the muscle used in the movement. That's why it's important not to begin exercise until instructed by your physician. Keep exercise moderate to ensure a positive effect on the healing process.

The Effect of Exercise on Immune Function

Increased immune function is another positive side effect of regular exercise. The increased oxygen intake from exercise enables your body to produce more immune cells, improves the function of those cells, and provides a much stronger defense for you against illness. If your immune system is like a coat of armor, then each exercise session could be likened to polishing that coat of armor. This is especially important for new moms whose immune function could be suppressed from fatigue and increased stress, as well as from passing some of their own immunity on to their baby through breast milk. Falling ill less often and recovering from illness faster will reduce your entire family's risk of spreading the germs and then succumbing to them. Many who exercise regularly find they get sick less often, and if or when they do, the time they are ill is shortened considerably.

A 2005 study, "The Effects of Exercise on the Immune System and Stress Hormones in Sportswomen," has shown the positive results of exercise: "Regular exercise has been reported to have several favorable effects on physiological, psychological, and immunologic functions, and increases the resistance against infections. Vigorous exercise, however, has been reported to have a negative effect on these functions."

The study compared sedentary women, aerobically active women (exercising moderately), and anaerobic women exercisers (those exercising intensely). The findings are quite impressive:

- The sedentary group showed levels of cortisol elevated by 31 percent and immunoglobulins (a large group of molecules containing carbohydrates and proteins that are secreted by plasma cells and function as antibodies) decreased by 30 percent.
- Women exercising at a moderate intensity were found to have increased their immunoglobulins for up to four days postexercise session as well as decreased their cortisol levels for two days postexercise.
- Women exercising intensely showed a slight decrease (less than 5 percent) in immunoglobulins as well as a very slight decrease (less than 1 percent) in cortisol levels.

"We conclude that regular and moderate exercise has favorable effects on the immune system by increasing immunoglobulins, which are potent protective factors," the study's authors write. Most busy moms will tell you that Mom getting sick is not an option. And while regular exercise might decrease your free time by 15 to 30 minutes a day, it is still far less time when you think about being down and out for an entire week with the flu. An ounce of prevention . . . .

Hormone Balance

Although we've already discussed many important reasons to exercise, I personally found the effects of exercise on hormone production, and in turn my mood and depression, to be very eye-opening. If no other reason resonates with you, maybe this one will!

Subcutaneous fat cells are responsible for producing 19 different hormones in women, including estrogen and progesterone. While maternal fat stores are important for maintaining proper hormone production and adequate milk supply, carrying too much body fat can result in an overproduction of many hormones, greatly increasing a woman's risk of cancer, especially breast, ovarian, endometrial, and cervical cancers. According to the American Council on Exercise, healthy body fat percentages are as follows:

GENERAL BODY FAT PERCENTAGE CATEGORIES		
Classification	**Women (% fat)**	**Men (% fat)**
Essential fat	10–12%	2–4%
Athletes	14–20%	6–13%
Fitness	21–24%	14–17%
Acceptable	25–31%	18–25%
Obese	32% plus	25% plus

Helping women maintain a healthy body fat to weight ratio and thus increasing the likelihood that their hormone production will be properly regulated are two reasons why doctors encourage women to exercise regularly. Both cardiovascular exercise and weight training play an important role in weight/body fat management. It is important for you to equate exercise to risk of disease reduction and to equate risk of certain diseases with hormone production.

If a doctor told you there was a way to reduce the risk of disease by 40 percent in your children by following some relatively simple steps, you would do it in a heartbeat. You would not make excuses, you would not wait, and you would not sit idly by. Yet, you often do wait, make excuses, and allow your risk of disease to increase. Reducing your risk is part of being the best mom you can be, and you are increasing the likelihood that you will be there to care for your children as they enter parenthood and all the challenges that come with it.

Depression: The Baby Blues and Beyond

A lot of people have heard about postpartum depression, but they don't know how it "looks" in real life. Here's my story about the days and weeks following my second child's birth.

PPD from the Inside

The first few weeks after Miles's birth were emotionally difficult at best. Mazie had recently experienced febrile seizures, which seemed to consume all of our thoughts and much of our time. While we received the best news we felt possible as to the reason for her seizures, the emotional toll was beginning to set in for me.

For three days, Miles and I bonded at the hospital, and although Eric and our families did visit and celebrate his birth, it was a much different atmosphere from Mazie's birth and homecoming. Not only did the fear of Mazie's seizures have a grip on me, but with most of our family helping to care for her while I cared for Miles, I also felt isolated and very depressed.

Sleep deprivation and plummeting hormones did nothing but make matters worse. I just wanted to crawl under the covers and never come out. I was embarrassed by what I thought was self-pity and never told a soul. I would wait until that glorious moment each day, or every other day, when I could grab a shower, and that is where I let it all out. I cried, I trembled, I allowed myself to feel what I didn't want to admit I was feeling. I couldn't stand the way I looked or felt. I kept thinking, "Why do other moms seem to have it all together and I am a *total* wreck? Why am I so bad at this?"

Luckily for me I was recovering from my second C-section faster than the first and was cleared for exercise after three weeks. Each night I placed my screaming little guy Miles (thanks to the colic, he screamed every night from 9 P.M. to midnight) in the stroller and headed out for a walk. It was late fall/early winter, and the chilly air energized me in minutes, and thankfully calmed him. I was also thankful for the darkness, as no one saw the tears running down my face with each and every step, each and every night. Without the hot showers and the cold night air, I do not know how I would have made it through.

I know now I suffered from postpartum depression, but at the time, I assumed I was just not meant to be a mom, or at least not the kind of mom I wanted to be. Almost three years later, I know that being more open about it would have served my family and my marriage better. My husband had no clue how badly I felt about myself, how I felt I had failed Mazie, that I felt my body had failed me, and how these issues impaired my ability to confide in my spouse. During this time, Eric and

I started to grow apart, and our friendship and intimacy waned. Luckily for us, we are now in a much better place, finally sleeping through the night, exercising on a regular basis, and confiding our feelings (big and small) in each other so that together we can strive to maintain balance in ourselves, our marriage, and parenthood.

Talk to Your Doctor!

One of the most important lessons that I learned through all of this is that ignoring something or trying to suppress it will only make it worse in the end! Postpartum depression is not a flaw. It is not the result of weakness, and it is not indicative of failure. In fact, it is a common side effect of motherhood. While exercise and lifestyle choices can lessen the symptoms of depression, first and foremost, talk to your doctor. If he or she is not an expert, they can no doubt point you to an expert in the field who can help you strategize on how to overcome your feelings. The sooner you manage and overcome depression, the sooner you will be the kind of mom you dreamt of being!

I love this quote. It has become my daily mantra: "Challenges make life interesting. Overcoming them gives life meaning."

Just like with other illnesses and diseases, early prevention can greatly diminish the recovery time and alleviate the symptoms of depression. According to staff at the Mayo Clinic, the following symptoms and feelings are considered "normal" baby blues, and may last for a few days after the birth:

- Mood swings
- Anxiety
- Sadness
- Irritability
- Crying

- Decreased concentration
- Trouble sleeping

Those suffering from postpartum depression, on the other hand, may experience the following symptoms for as little as a few weeks and as long as up to a year post-childbirth.

- Loss of appetite
- Insomnia
- Intense irritability and anger
- Overwhelming fatigue
- Loss of interest in sex
- Lack of joy in life
- Feelings of shame, guilt, or inadequacy
- Severe mood swings
- Difficulty bonding with the baby
- Withdrawal from family and friends
- Thoughts of harming yourself or the baby

Isolation can increase the feelings of postpartum depression. Talk to your doctor openly about your feelings and symptoms. He or she is more than willing to help you, but your doctor is not a mind reader, and you need to help him or her help you.

Doctors are not the only resources for overcoming postpartum depression and/or the baby blues. Other moms who have been there or are there can be a tremendous support system. Exercise groups such as StrollerFit and its social group StrollerFriends can be life-changing. Bonding with other moms while reaping the benefits of exercise and reducing feelings of isolation result in a support system for new moms that can help them embrace all the challenges that motherhood presents.

How Exercise Can Help

A prescription of exercise to alleviate some of the symptoms of depression is increasingly in use by the medical community due to its powerful effects. Kristin Vickers-Douglas, PhD, a psychologist at Mayo Clinic, in Rochester, Minnesota, says, "It's not a magic bullet, but increasing physical activity is a positive and active strategy to help manage depression and anxiety."

For exercise to have an effect on mood and depression, it simply just has to be done. However it fits in to your day is how you should do it. Mood-altering exercise sessions can be as little as 10 to 15 minutes. While it is best to set a goal for 30 minutes a day, breaking that up into bits and pieces will not diminish the mood-altering effects. In fact, on atypically difficult days, exercising two to three times for 10 to 15 minutes each time can be extremely helpful in the dissipation of anxiety and stress.

Taking the First Steps Back

Now that you know many of the powerful benefits that exercise offers you, it is hard to sit by and not do it! However, for new moms, exercise can be difficult physically. Many moms will try to jump back into fitness wanting to shed the weight and feel like themselves again. Others will be too overwhelmed with their new mom schedules and too unfamiliar with their new mom bodies to try.

Easing into fitness following a C-section delivery is a must for the body, mind, and spirit. Right now, your body doesn't look familiar, because it isn't. It has gone through an incredible series of changes to create, sustain, and introduce new life to the world. I am sure that you, like most new moms, can rattle off more than a few ways in which your body has changed. You probably can't miss the changes that you see in the mirror, but understanding the changes beneath the skin will help you not only take the right approach to fitness but also help motivate you into taking action!

Why You Feel Weak

Like it or not, there is a certain amount of deconditioning that occurs in the average mom during pregnancy, even those exercising throughout. This detraining takes place both in the aerobic systems (heart and lungs) and in our muscular systems. For those with extreme circumstances such as bed rest or those unable to exercise during pregnancy, additional muscle loss and aerobic deconditioning can take place. Aerobic deconditioning often occurs in pregnancy due to a drop in intensity of exercise being performed as well as a decrease in the duration for which moms-to-be are exercising. Loss of muscular strength can also be attributed to changes in frequency, duration, and consistency of exercise routines, as fatigue, morning sickness, and possible other complications set in. According to a study called "Pregnancy-Related Changes in Physical Activity," muscular strength is lost both in the upper body and lower body, with the greatest loss found in the legs. One might think that the additional "load" on the muscles of the legs due to weight gain during pregnancy would keep them from losing strength—not so. The findings (loss of aerobic conditioning and muscular strength) are consistent in both women who remained active during pregnancy and those who did not.

Your Posture

Many physical changes also occur to your posture as pregnancy progresses. It is important that you reverse these changes, as they can lead to increased muscular fatigue and injury. Many postpartum discomforts (such as lingering back and leg pain and joint discomfort) can be attributed to the postural changes that occurred as the baby grew and the pregnancy progressed. These changes affect many areas of the body, causing certain muscles to become overworked and tight while the opposing muscles are overstretched and weakened. Changes to the hip and shoulder joints as well as the abdominal wall and pelvic floor must be addressed in a postpartum exercise program in order to alleviate poor posture and return the body to proper form and function. Here are some common changes in posture due to pregnancy. First, the forward tilt of the pelvis (lordosis) causes:

- Pubic bone and tailbone to move backward
- Overarching of the low back
- Shortening of the hip flexors, resulting in chronic tightness
- Tightening of the quadratus lumborum (lower back muscles)
- Overstretching of the hamstrings
- Weakening of the glutes
- Rounding forward of the shoulders (kyphosis), which causes shortening and tightening of the pectoral (chest) muscles
- Overstretching and weakening serratus anterior and trapezius (upper back muscles)
- Collapsing of the chest, weakening of the intercostals muscles (which are found between the ribs and aid in proper breathing)
- Jutting forward of the head

In addition, poor pregnancy posture can lead to:

- Compression on the vertebral discs
- Ligament strain/joint discomfort

- Improper use of muscles causing soreness and fatigue
- Reduction of lung capacity
- Strain of the mid back and neck
- Back pain and fatigue
- Loss of height

These changes lead to improper muscular use. Poor pregnancy posture does not fade away after the baby is born. In fact, many moms find themselves in this same posture years down the line. Poor posture affects everything from decreasing the amount of oxygen you breathe in and your ability to expel toxins through exhales to the way you carry your baby on your hip or in your arms.

Your body's main postural muscles (found in the abdominals, back, hips, shoulders, and neck) are those most affected by pregnancy. This is what leaves you incapable of proper posture and increases your risk of injury as well as robs you of much-needed energy. When one group of muscles is not doing its job properly, another group must pick up the slack, performing its own function and the function of the nonfunctioning group. Such is the case when your postural muscles are not returned to their original length through proper exercise. Suddenly your legs, which are meant to simply mobilize you, now must work to stabilize you and then mobilize you. Because your leg muscles are the largest in the body, they use the most energy. This misuse of the muscles will lead to fatigue. The problem for most new moms is that your core muscles have been overstretched for so many months that not only are they the wrong length but they have also forgotten what their jobs are due to a lack of proper use! In the chapters to come, we will address each of these changes, reminding your body to properly stabilize itself.

Look for Specific Postnatal Exercise Routines

It doesn't seem quite fair that as your level of responsibility shoots through the roof when parenthood begins, your bodies are functioning at less than an optimal level. Though they're challenging to overcome, each change is reversible and you can attain noticeable increases in strength and aerobic fitness as well as improved posture in a few short weeks. Patience is an important part of the process in regaining your fitness and your quest to fit into those prepregnancy jeans. Remember, it took ten months for your body to ready you and your baby for delivery, and it will take a number of months to change it back!

It is vital to your success in reclaiming your body that you participate in an exercise program that has been designed specifically for the stage of life you are in and one that addresses the changes to your body and lifestyle. This means that the group fitness classes and the at-home fitness DVDs that you did prior to pregnancy are not suitable for you now. Even though you're no longer pregnant, you're still dealing with the effects of hormones; ligament, tendon, and muscular changes; energy usage; and changing emotional needs. Proper exercise programming for every stage of motherhood will not only help you adhere to the exercise program but also promote health and well-being for your entire family, raise your self-esteem, increase your fitness, and give you the energy to make it through every day.

The Science Behind a Postnatal Exercise Program

The hormone relaxin is one of the main reasons for a specific exercise program. Up to 10 times the normal amount of relaxin is found in the body during pregnancy. Its job is to soften the connective tissues in your body, allowing the pelvis to properly widen for delivery. Unfortunately for moms, relaxin affects every joint in the body, and it often brings with it inflammation and discomfort. A mom's tendons and ligaments will not be as capable of protecting the joints during activity in the postpartum period due to increased levels of relaxin.

It can take a full *four* months for relaxin levels to return to normal postpartum. During this period, avoid any and all fast stops and starts and quick side-to-side movements, and avoid (or at least take extreme caution during) explosive movements while exercising as well. Plyometrics, jump squats, and even soccer or tennis can potentially cause damage to the knee and hip joints during this period. The widening of the hips for delivery creates a large Q angle, the angle at which the femur (upper leg bone) meets the tibia (lower leg bone). The greater this angle is, the higher the risk of knee injuries, ranging from tendonitis to damage or tears of the anterior cruciate ligament (ACL). A proper postnatal exercise program will address the changes to the hips as well as other bone structure and soft tissue changes.

What Is Diastasis Recti?

A postnatal-specific program will also take into consideration the possibility of diastasis recti, a separation between the left and right side of the rectus abdominis muscle. Again, the hormone relaxin comes into play as it softens the linea alba (line of connective tissue that connects the two halves of the rectus abdominis—the "six-pack muscle") as well. The softening of this tissue along with pressure from a growing baby causes a separation of the two halves. What is important to know is that abdominal muscle separation along the linea alba of more than 2.5 fingers wide can increase pelvic instability and increase low back pain. For this reason, proper abdominal training is a must. It is most important to know if you have a separation that is wider than 2.5 fingers so that you can avoid moves that could put you at risk for back or hip injury. Avoid moves that involve twisting and curving the spine at the same time until the separation is less than 2.5 fingers. Moms should also avoid backbends (even over an exercise ball) and hard crunching or shortening of the six-pack muscle (traditional situps). I had a 3.5-finger separation but with proper core training (which you have in this book!), I was able to reduce the separation and within a few short months postpregnancy was back to normal! Once the transversus abdominis is returned to proper strength, length, and function (through the exercises found in this book) you will be free to move without restriction.

For more information on diastasis recti, visit *www.befitmom.com*. You will find common misconceptions and other valuable information here, as well as this test for diastasis recti:

- Lie on your back with your knees bent and the soles of your feet on the floor.
- Place one hand behind your head, and the other hand on your abdomen, with your fingertips across your midline—parallel with your waistline—at the level of your bellybutton.
- With your abdominal wall relaxed, gently press your fingertips into your abdomen.
- Roll your upper body off the floor into a "crunch," making sure that your ribcage moves closer to your pelvis.
- Move your fingertips back and forth across your midline, feeling for the right and left sides of your rectus abdominis muscle.

Special Advice for Moms Who Are Breastfeeding

Relaxin levels will remain higher in postnatal women who are breastfeeding. Avoiding the abovementioned movements will be necessary to prevent injury for the entire time breastfeeding occurs and for four weeks thereafter. For moms who are breastfeeding, there are a few others items to take into consideration as well! Take comfort that moderate exercise does not interfere with milk production; in some cases exercise has been shown to increase production slightly, as long as fluid needs for mom are being met. The American College of Sports Medicine recommends drinking 8 to 10 ounces of fluid for every 15 minutes of exercise. Keeping up with fluid intake is also important as it aids in regulating body temperature, proper digestion, delivery of oxygen and nutrients to every cell in the body, and the removal of toxins.

Many moms are also concerned that exercise will change the taste of breast milk due to an increase in lactic acid from exercise. While lactic acid (a byproduct of carbohydrates that is broken down as fuel for exercise) production does increase during exercise, maintaining a level of exertion below 80 percent of your maximum ability will not adversely affect the taste of the milk produced during or after the exercise session. However, your skin may be more salty than desired by your little one due to sweat; a quick shower or wipe down can alleviate this condition.

When to Start "Regular" Exercising Again

The length of time for which a new mom should participate in a postnatal exercise program before returning to "regular" exercise will be different for each woman and each pregnancy. Personally, I bounced back better after my second child and felt stronger sooner, but the weight took longer to come off. The length of time to participate in a specific postnatal program is also dependent on the circumstances that took place during pregnancy and delivery. Moms of multiples should expect their bodies to take a bit longer to bounce back, as they underwent more change and have a greater expenditure of energy in caring for two or more babies, and moms who were restricted from exercise during pregnancy will also experience a longer rebound. I highly recommend that you participate in postnatal exercise programs for a minimum of 16 weeks, starting from the date your doctor clears you for exercise.

Moms who are breastfeeding should stay in postnatal fitness programs for at least one month past the date that weaning takes place. It is important to note that some of the pregnancy/postpartum changes can take up to 18 months to alleviate or reverse. During this entire 18-month period, your risk of injury remains higher. I instruct my clients to follow a postnatal-specific workout plan until 18 months after their last child is born; this way, I know they are in good hands and receiving specialized care.

Postnatal Exercise Program
Months One, Two, and Three: Restorative Health and Well-Being

After you are cleared for exercise, the concentration will be on core strength, restoring proper posture, muscular length, and joint stabilization through biweekly strength training sessions. Walk or ride on a stationary bike two to three times a week for 20 to 30 minutes to improve cardiovascular efficiency and speed the healing process.

Month one begins when you are cleared for exercise from your doctor and not a minute before! The workouts listed below are described in detail in the coming chapters.

MONTHS ONE, TWO, AND THREE: RESTORATIVE HEALTH AND WELL-BEING					
	Stretches	Cardio	Core	Upper Body	Lower Body
Month 1	Perform all stretches in Chapter 3 daily	25 minutes at 65% effort 3× per week	A 2× per week (3× if energy allows)	A	A
Month 2	Perform all stretches in Chapter 3 daily	30 minutes at 65% effort 3× per week	B 2× per week (3× if energy allows)	B	B
Month 3	Perform all stretches in Chapter 3 daily	35 minutes at 70% effort 3× per week	C 2× per week (3× if energy allows)	C	C

Months Four, Five, and Six: Gaining Strength and Stability

With a continued focus on core strength, you will begin to add movement to the resistance training exercises preparing your body for the physical challenges of motherhood. You will also begin working to restore a sense of balance, which can be thrown off during pregnancy and in the first few months of motherhood. Through an increase in the duration of cardiovascular exercise your endurance will begin to improve (stick to the golden rule of not adding more than 10 percent per week in total weekly minutes of exercise).

MONTHS FOUR, FIVE, AND SIX: GAINING STRENGTH AND STABILITY					
	Stretches	Cardio	Core	Upper Body	Lower Body
Month 4	Perform all stretches in Chapter 3 3× per week	30 minutes at 70–75% effort 3× per week	D 2× per week (3× if energy allows)	D	D
Month 5	Perform all stretches in Chapter 3 3× per week	35 minutes at 70–75% effort 4× per week	E 2× per week C 1× per week	E	E
Month 6	Perform all stretches in Chapter 3 3× per week	35 minutes at 70–75% effort 4× per week	F 2× per week C 1× per week	F	F

Months Seven, Eight, and Nine: Increase Cardiovascular Performance

In addition to taking on more challenging core work, you can now slightly increase the intensity of your cardiovascular exercise. You can also increase the number of repetitions for strength training moves. This phase will improve your cardiovascular endurance and you will find yourself more capable of resisting fatigue.

MONTHS SEVEN, EIGHT, AND NINE: INCREASE CARDIOVASCULAR PERFORMANCE				
	Stretches	Cardio	Core	Total Body
Month 7	Perform all stretches in Chapter 3 3× per week	40 minutes at 70–75% effort 4× per week	G 1× per week	A 2× per week
Month 8	Perform all stretches in Chapter 3 3× per week	40 minutes at 70–75% effort 4× per week	H 1× per week	B 2× per week
Month 9	Perform all stretches in Chapter 3 3× per week	40 minutes at 70–75% effort 4× per week	I 1× per week	C 2× per week

Months Ten, Eleven, and Twelve: Increasing Muscular Endurance

As your baby continues to grow, the load on your muscles can begin to take a toll. No doubt you are carrying 20 to 40 pounds up and down the steps, and to the car and back a dozen times a day. Through proper muscular conditioning, you can reduce fatigue and gain energy that allows you to stay on your toes and be active for more hours each day (and chase a baby on the move!).

MONTHS TEN, ELEVEN, AND TWELVE: INCREASING MUSCULAR ENDURANCE				
	Stretches	Cardio	Core	Total Body
Month 10	Perform all stretches in Chapter 3 3× per week	45 minutes at 75% effort 4× per week	J 2× per week C 1× per week	D 2× per week
Month 11	Perform all stretches in Chapter 3 3× per week	40 minutes at 75–80% effort 4× per week	I 2× per week C 1× per week	E 2× per week
Month 12	Perform all stretches in Chapter 3 3× per week	40 minutes at 75–80% effort 4× per week	J 2× per week C 1× per week	F 2× per week

Months Thirteen Through Eighteen: Owning Your Body

As your risk of injury begins to decrease and your confidence begins to soar, your body becomes your own again. Keeping up with a toddler is tough work, and your workouts must increase in difficulty so that your mom life doesn't break you down. An increased level of difficulty can be achieved simply by changing one thing about the way you are working out. Expect higher heart rates as well as being put off-balance so that your body gains more balance! Simple, small changes add up to big results!

MONTHS THIRTEEN THROUGH EIGHTEEN: OWNING YOUR BODY				
	Stretches	Cardio	Core	Total Body
Month 13	Perform all stretches in Chapter 3 3× per week	10 minutes at 75% effort, 10 minutes at 80%, 5 minutes at 85%, and 5 minutes at 75% 1× per week & 40 minutes at 75–80% effort 3× per week	I 2× per week	G
Month 14	Perform all stretches in Chapter 3 3× per week	10 minutes at 75% effort, 10 minutes at 80%, 10 minutes at 85%, and 5 minutes at 75% 1× per week & 40 minutes at 75–80% effort 3× per week	J 2× per week C 1× per week	H
Months 15–16	Perform all stretches in Chapter 3 3× per week	10 minutes at 75% effort, 10 minutes at 80%, 15 minutes at 85%, and 5 minutes at 75% 1× per week & 40 minutes at 75–80% effort 3× per week	I 2× per week C 1× per week	I
Months 17–18	Perform all stretches in Chapter 3 3× per week	10 minutes at 75% effort, 10 minutes at 80%, 20 minutes at 85%, and 5 minutes at 75% 1× per week & 40 minutes at 75–80% effort 3× per week	J 2× per week C 1× per week	J

Why Weight Training Is Important

Strength training, also known as resistance training or weight training, is vital to feeling good, remaining injury-free, boosting bone strength, improving posture, and losing/maintaining weight. Over the years, I have found that most women don't mind cardiovascular conditioning. Cardio is most easily worked into the day for new moms. After all, babies love the outdoors, and pushing them in a stroller feels like we are doing something for them and for us. Unfortunately, many women do not enjoy weight training as much as going for a walk in the sunshine. Go figure!

However, without weight training, your body will pay a price for the physical demands of motherhood, and your metabolism will slow as you age, making weight gain unavoidable.

For the first few weeks, the goal of strength training and core training is simply to regain stability and correct the structural damage (poor posture) that pregnancy created. These gentle moves will increase the blood flow, aid the muscles in returning to their proper length, and begin to build lean muscle. While the end result of strength training is increased fat burning, the action of weight training burns carbohydrates. It is the rapid use of carbohydrates (and the subsequent overload of pyruvic acid as the carbohydrate is broken down) that causes a burning sensation in the muscle during the actual movement. It is also the reason for feeling sore in the 24 to 48 hours after strength training.

This soreness (Delayed Onset Muscle Soreness, or DOMS) should be moderate and should not last more than 72 hours after the strength training activity. Extreme soreness or soreness that lasts longer than 72 hours may signify injury. This program has been constructed to give strength and stability with minimal soreness and very low risk of injury. Keep in mind that too much soreness may interfere with your new life as a mom; therefore, this gentle routine is best. Once through this recovery period, your workouts can become more difficult; however, moderation is always best. If I had to pick a theme for these workouts, it would be just enough to gain strength but not enough to interfere with life!

Strength Training "Rules" for Success

- Do not hold your breath while you strength train. Exhale on the hard part (contraction), and inhale on the easy part (release).
- Give your body 48 hours of rest before strength training the same body part(s) again. For instance, do not perform leg strength training moves two days in a row.
- Eat protein and carbohydrates within 30 to 45 minutes of finishing your strength training to allow for muscle repair and growth, as well as sustained energy.
- Make sure that you have eaten 150 to 200 calories in the three hours prior to exercise to ensure you have the energy to complete the session.
- Work hard enough that you have to think about it, but not so hard that you use momentum or have to change your posture to complete the exercise.
- Increase repetitions or weight or resistance level every other week, but do not increase all at the same time.
- Be consistent! If you don't use it, you lose it.
- Do not try to make up for missed workouts! This will leave you too tired and crunched for time. If you miss one, just skip it altogether. If you miss two or more, when you get back on track, go back to the last workout you did do and start the program from there. Jumping to harder efforts will not bring results sooner; instead it will bring burnout, fatigue, and possibly injury.
- Rest between sets should be 30 to 90 seconds.
- If you begin to lose your form, rest! It is better to complete eight perfectly executed moves than twelve not-so-perfect ones. The not-so-perfect ones open the door to injury.

Don't Forget to Stretch!

Stretching should follow each and every workout and can even be done on days that you don't work out. It is best to stretch after the exercise is complete. At this time your body is warm and your muscles are more pliable. If stretching on a nonworkout day, take a warm bath or shower prior to stretching. In the midst of stretching, breathe deeply to relax your body, stretch to the point of tension but never pain, and hold the stretch for 20 seconds at a time. Refer back to Chapter 3 for pictures and descriptions of the necessary stretches.

UPPER BODY STRENGTH TRAINING

The Workouts

For these workouts, you will need a small squeezable ball (just a bit larger than a grapefruit) and a resistance tube. In the photos, I have used a figure 8 resistance tube as well as a standard resistance tube. As your body becomes stronger, it may be necessary to use hand weights in place of the resistance tube for more of a challenge. Begin with 5-pound weights and progress by 2 or 3 pounds as necessary. The workout should always be somewhat challenging!

Since the body learns by repetition, you will be repeating the same exercises for 4 weeks at a time. If you get to the end of the set (10 to 12 repetitions of the same exercise) and you are not somewhat challenged by it, it is time to increase the repetitions you are doing in each set. You can add 2 to 3 repetitions to each move to gently challenge the body when need be. If the instruction is to hold a movement for 15 to 30 seconds and the time frame is not somewhat challenging, add 10 to 15 seconds to the move to signal to your body that it is time to grow stronger.

The ★ symbol before the name of an exercise is to inform you that this is a new exercise to be added onto the prior group of exercises.

UPPER BODY A

- **Seated Isometric Chest Press:** 15-second press, rest, and repeat for a total of three sets
- **Seated Isometric Biceps Ball Press:** 15-second press, rest, and repeat for a total of three sets

UPPER BODY B

- **Seated Isometric Chest Press:** 20-second press, rest, and repeat
- **Seated Isometric Biceps Ball Press:** 20-second press, rest, and repeat for a total of three sets
- ***Seated Rear Delt Row:** three sets of 10 repetitions
- ***Upright Row with Oblique Crunch:** three sets of 10 repetitions
- ***Triceps Dip:** two sets of 8 dips

UPPER BODY C

- **Seated Isometric Chest Press:** 25-second press, rest, and repeat for a total of three sets
- **Seated Isometric Biceps Ball Press:** 25-second press, rest, and repeat for a total of three sets
- **Seated Rear Delt Row:** three sets of 12–15 repetitions
- **Upright Row with Oblique Crunch:** three sets of 12–15 repetitions
- **Triceps Dip:** three sets of 12–15 repetitions

UPPER BODY D

- ***Modified Push-up:** two sets of 10
- **Upright Row with Oblique Crunch:** three sets of 12–15
- ***Rear Delt Fly:** three sets of 10
- ***Biceps Curl:** two sets of 10
- **Triceps Dip:** three sets of 10

UPPER BODY E
- **Modified Push-up:** three sets of 10
- **Upright Row with Oblique Crunch:** three sets of 12
- **Rear Delt Fly:** three sets of 10
- **Biceps Curl:** three sets of 12
- **Triceps Dip:** three sets of 10

BICEPS CURL

Stand on a resistance tube with your feet shoulder-distance apart, very slight bend in your knee. Begin with your hands by your hips, holding the handle of a tube in each hand. Exhale as you lift your hands up, keeping your elbows at your sides. Lower your hands back down slowly and repeat.

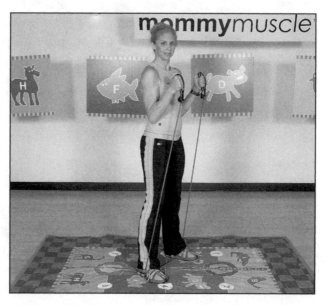

▲   BICEPS CURL

MODIFIED PUSH-UP

Come down to the floor, on your knees, and walk your hands out in front of you. Place them on the floor, wider than your shoulders. Keep your knees bent on the ground and your feet in the air. Keeping your body straight (no bend in the hips), lower down into the push-up position. Make sure your elbows are over your wrists to protect your joints from too much pressure. Do not let your back sag; keep your navel pulled back toward your spine. Inhale as you lower; exhale as you press away from the mat.

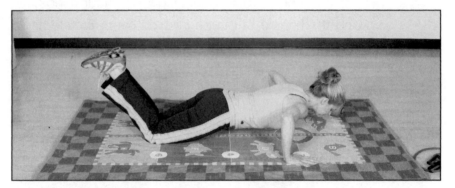

▲ MODIFIED PUSH-UP

REAR DELT FLY

Wrap a resistance tube around each hand, letting the handles fall off to the sides and leaving some slack in the tube between your hands (Figure 1). With your arms straight, but elbows not locked, exhale and pull your arms away from each other (Figure 2). Squeeze between your shoulder blades and pause briefly, then release slowly back to the starting position.

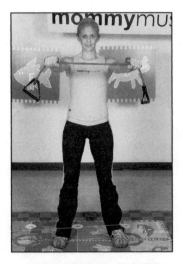 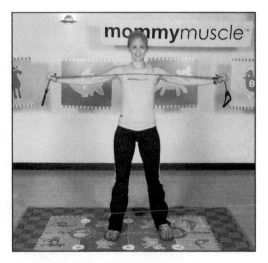

▲ REAR DELT FLY, FIGURE 1   ▲   REAR DELT FLY, FIGURE 2

SEATED ISOMETRIC BICEPS BALL PRESS

Place a small ball in between your biceps and your forearm on each arm. Press your hands down toward your shoulders, squeezing the balls. Hold for 15 seconds, then rest.

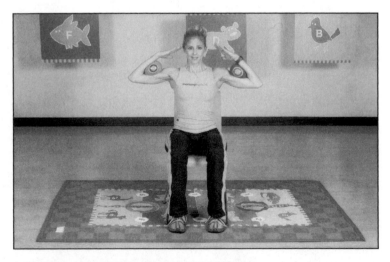

▲ SEATED ISOMETRIC BICEPS BALL PRESS

SEATED ISOMETRIC CHEST PRESS

Place a small ball between your hands. Keep your elbows out, and fingertips pointing up. Press the palms of your hands in toward each other. Hold for 15 seconds, then rest.

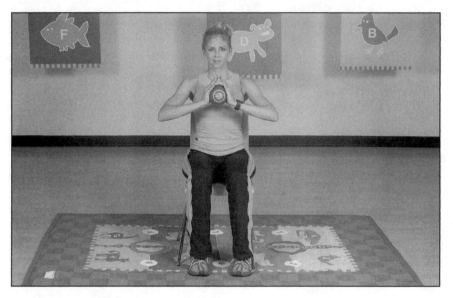

▲ SEATED ISOMETRIC CHEST PRESS

SEATED REAR DELT ROW

Place the resistance tube around the arch of one foot. If the tube has two handles, hold one in each hand. If not, hold the loop in both hands. Sit up tall, and draw your navel back to your spine (Figure 1). Pull your elbows back, tightening the resistance on the tube (Figure 2). Squeeze your shoulder blades back and down; hold for 3 seconds. Release and repeat. Inhale on the release, exhale on the pull.

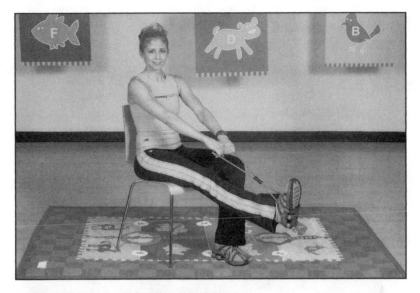

▲ SEATED REAR DELT ROW, FIGURE 1

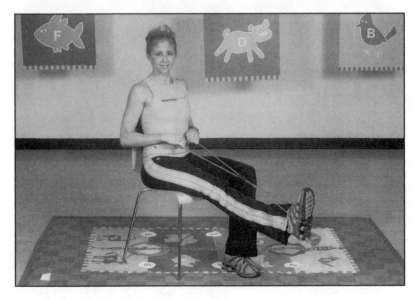

▲ SEATED REAR DELT ROW, FIGURE 2

TRICEPS DIP

Sit on the floor, feet hip-distance apart and hands placed at your sides. Your thumbs should be resting as close to your hips as possible, with fingertips pointing toward your toes. Straighten your arms, lifting your hips off the floor. Do not lock your elbow joint. Bend at your elbow, bringing your hips closer to the floor (but not touching!). Exhale and press away from the floor, then repeat.

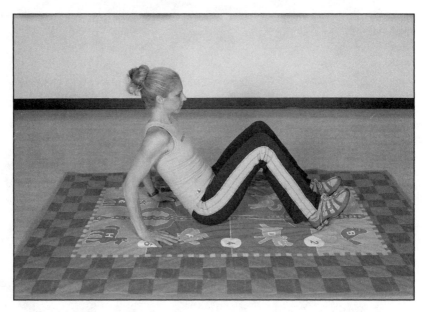

▲ TRICEPS DIP

UPRIGHT ROW WITH OBLIQUE CRUNCH

Seated in a chair, secure the resistance tube under the arch of your right foot. Hold the other end in your right hand. Draw your elbow up to the ceiling as you tilt your shoulders and reach your left hand's fingertips toward the floor, near your left foot, pause briefly. Return to an upright position, and then slowly release the tension out of the resistance tube.

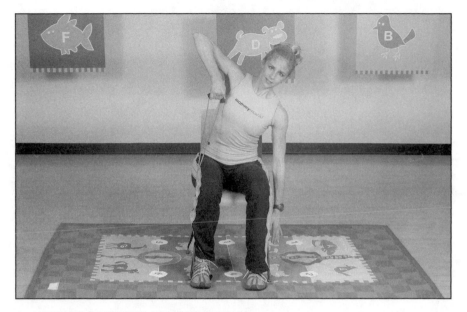

▲ UPRIGHT ROW WITH OBLIQUE CRUNCH

LOWER BODY STRENGTH TRAINING

The Workouts

For these workouts, you will need a small squeezable ball (just a bit larger than a grapefruit) and a resistance tube. In the photos, I have used a figure 8 resistance tube as well as a standard resistance tube. As your body becomes stronger, it may be necessary to use hand weights in place of the resistance tube for more of a challenge. Begin with 5-pound weights and progress by 2 or 3 pounds as necessary. The workout should always be somewhat challenging!

Since the body learns by repetition, you will be repeating the same exercises for four weeks at a time. If you get to the end of the set (10 to 12 repetitions of the same exercise) and you are not somewhat challenged by it, it is time to increase the repetitions you are doing in each set. You can add 2 to 3 repetitions to each move to gently challenge the body when need be. If the instruction is to hold a movement for 15 to 30 seconds and the time frame is not somewhat challenging, add 10 to 15 seconds to the move to signal to your body that it is time to grow stronger.

The ★ symbol before the name of an exercise is to inform you that this is a new exercise to be added onto the prior group of exercises.

LOWER BODY A

- **Inner Thigh Squeeze:** three sets of 10-second holds
- **Wall Squat:** three sets of 10-second holds
- **Leg Extension:** three sets of 10, each leg
- **Calf Raise:** three sets of 10

LOWER BODY B

- **Inner Thigh Squeeze:** three sets of 10-second holds
- **Wall Squat:** three sets of 15-second holds
- **Leg Extension:** three sets of 10, each leg
- **Calf Raise:** three sets of 10
- ***Side Lying Leg Lifts:** two sets of 10, each leg
- ***Hip Circles:** two sets of 10, each leg

LOWER BODY C

- **Wall Squat:** three sets of 30-second holds
- **Leg Extension:** three sets of 12–15, each leg
- **Calf Raise:** three sets of 12–15
- **Side Lying Leg Lifts:** three sets of 12–15, each leg
- **Hip Circles:** three sets of 12, each leg

LOWER BODY D

- ***Pliéd Squat:** two sets of 10
- ***Stationary Lunge:** two sets of 10 each leg
- **Calf Raise:** three sets of 12; add 3–5-lb hand weights to increase difficulty
- ***Glute Press:** two sets of 10, each leg

LOWER BODY E

- **Pliéd Squat:** three sets of 10–12
- **Stationary Lunge:** three sets of 10–12, each leg

- **Calf Raise:** three sets of 12–15 (with hand weights)
- **Glute Press:** three sets of 12–15

LOWER BODY F

- **Pliéd Squat:** three sets of 15
- **Stationary Lunge:** three sets of 12–15, each leg
- **Calf Raise:** three sets of 12–15 (with hand weights)
- **Glute Press:** three sets of 12–15

CALF RAISE

Stand behind a sturdy chair, placing your fingers on the back of the chair to aid in balance (Figure 1). Point your toes outward, creating a wide angle. Lift up on your toes, without pulling back on the chair (Figure 2). Squeeze your calf muscles, hold for 3 seconds, and release. Inhale as you lower, exhale as you lift. Keep your navel pulled back toward your spine, your chin lifted, and your shoulders back.

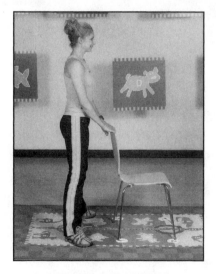
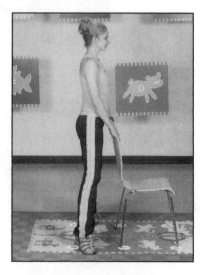

▲ CALF RAISE, FIGURE 1   ▲ CALF RAISE, FIGURE 2

GLUTE PRESS

Get on all fours on the floor or an exercise mat. Place a resistance tube behind your right foot, in the arch of your shoe. Hold the handles of the tube under your hands. Exhale as you press your leg back behind you; inhale as you slowly release.

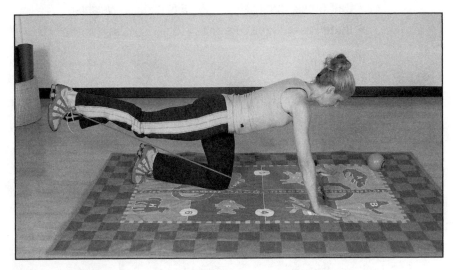

▲ GLUTE PRESS

HIP CIRCLES

Get in an all-fours position with your hands directly under your shoulders. Place a small squeezable ball behind your right knee and apply gentle pressure to the ball, keeping it in place. Lift your right knee off the floor, then press your foot toward your glutes while lifting your knee out to the side (think dog + fire hydrant!). Lower back to the start. Repeat these circles 12 times, then switch legs.

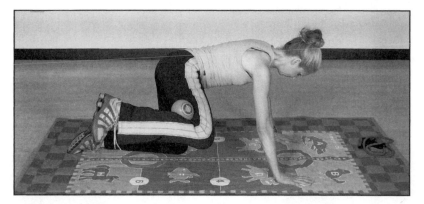

▲ HIP CIRCLES

INNER THIGH SQUEEZE

Place a small ball between your knees. Sit up tall and pull navel toward your spine. Press your knees toward each other and hold for 10 seconds. Remember to breathe!

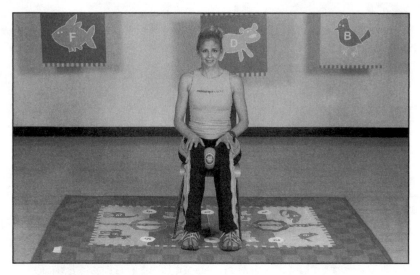

▲ INNER THIGH SQUEEZE

LEG EXTENSION

Sit in a sturdy, nonplush chair. Place the resistance tube in the arch of your left foot, bending your leg at a 90 degree angle (Figure 1). Keep your other foot flat on the floor. Hold the other end(s) of the tube in your hands. Sit up tall, with navel pulled to spine. Exhale as you unbend your left leg out away from you (Figure 2). Do not lock your knee joint; keep a very slight bend in the knee. Hold for a moment, release with an inhale, and repeat.

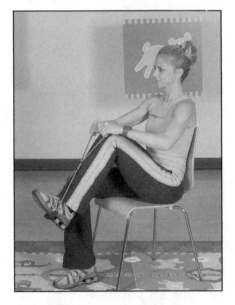

▲ LEG EXTENSION, FIGURE 1

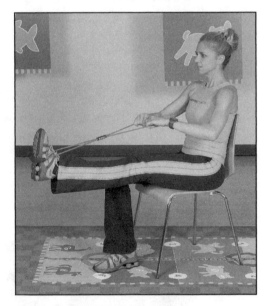

▲ LEG EXTENSION, FIGURE 2

PLIÉD SQUAT

Step your feet out wider than your shoulders, and turn your toes out slightly. Bring your closed fists together near your navel. Inhale as you lower down just like you are about to sit in a chair. Exhale as you press through your heels and return to a standing position. Keep your shoulders back over your hips, chin lifted, and do not allow your knees to move out over your toes at any time during the squat.

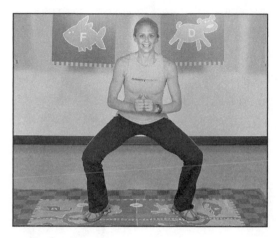

▲ PLIÉD SQUAT

SIDE LYING LEG LIFTS

Lie on your right side, body in a straight line. Exhale as you lift your top leg up; hold for 3 seconds and release the leg back down, but do not rest it on the other one. Repeat 10 times, rest, and repeat again before switching to the other side. The leg only needs to lift a few inches; if you take the leg too high, it will cause you to bend in the hips or rotate your leg—avoid those things.

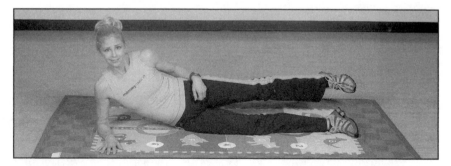

▲ SIDE LYING LEG LIFTS

STATIONARY LUNGE

Begin in a standing position. Step your right foot out in front of you, and bend at the knee, dropping into a lunge. Make sure your right knee stays in line with your right ankle at a 90 degree angle. Keep your shoulders back and your chin lifted. Inhale as you lower. On the exhale, press through your right heel and straighten your legs without locking your knee joint. Complete a set of 10 on this side, and then switch legs.

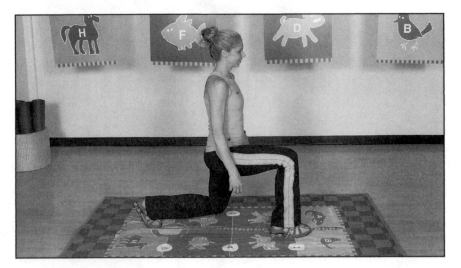

▲ STATIONARY LUNGE

WALL SQUAT

Stand in front of a wall (facing away from it), with your feet hip-distance apart and one or two steps away from the wall. Reach your hands back to the wall to help balance yourself (Figure 1). Lower down into a squat and remove your hands from the wall (Figure 2). Make sure your knees are not jutting out over your toes; instead "stack the joints" (knee over the ankle). Pull your navel back toward your spine. Pull your shoulders back toward the wall and keep your chin lifted. Breathe deeply. Count to 10 (slowly), then place your hands back on the wall and return to standing.

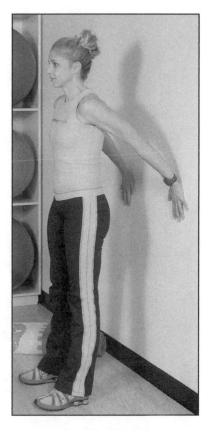

▲ WALL SQUAT, FIGURE 1

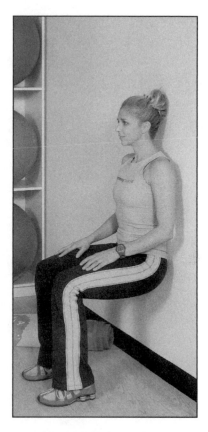

▲ WALL SQUAT, FIGURE 2

CORE STRENGTH TRAINING

The Workouts

For these workouts, you will need a small squeezable ball (just a bit larger than a grapefruit) and a resistance tube. In the photos, I have used a standard resistance tube.

Since the body learns by repetition, you will be repeating the same exercises for four weeks at a time. If you get to the end of the set (10 to 12 repetitions of the same exercise) and you are not somewhat challenged by it, it is time to increase the repetitions you are doing in each set. You can add 2 to 3 repetitions to each move to gently challenge the body when need be. If the instruction is to hold a movement for 15 to 30 seconds and the time frame is not somewhat challenging, add 10 to 15 seconds to the move to signal to your body that it is time to grow stronger.

The ★ symbol before the name of an exercise is to inform you that this is a new exercise to be added onto the prior group of exercises.

CORE A

- **Compression:** three sets, 10 inhales and exhales
- **Abdominal Compression with Leg Lift:** two sets each leg, 10 breaths each time
- **Tabletop with Ball Squeeze:** two sets, 15-second hold each time
- **Tabletop with Head Lift:** two sets of 15-second holds
- **Bridge:** three sets of 15-second holds
- **Modified Side Plank:** two sets of 10-second holds on each side

CORE B

- **Compression:** three sets, 10 inhales and exhales
- **Abdominal Compression with Leg Lift:** two sets each leg, 10 breaths each time
- **Tabletop with Ball Squeeze:** two sets, 15-second hold each time
- **Tabletop with Head Lift:** two sets of 15-second holds
- **Bridge:** three sets of 15-second holds
- **Modified Side Plank:** two sets each side, 10-second hold
- ***Ball Squeeze Between Ankles:** two sets of 10-second holds each

CORE C

- ***Compression with Ball Squeeze:** three sets, 10 inhales and exhales
- **Abdominal Compression with Leg Lift:** three sets each leg, 10 breaths each time
- **Tabletop with Ball Squeeze:** two sets, 15-second hold each
- **Tabletop with Head Lift:** two sets, 15-second hold each
- **Bridge:** three sets of 15-second holds
- **Modified Side Plank:** three sets each side, 10-second hold

CORE D

- **Tabletop with Ball Squeeze:** two sets of 15-second holds
- **Tabletop with Head Lift:** two sets of 10 crunches

- ***Tabletop with Heel Touch:** two sets of 5 each leg
- ***Leg Lift with Flat Band:** two sets of 10-second holds
- ***Superman:** two sets of 10-second holds
- ***Modified Plank:** two sets of 10-second holds
- **Modified Side Plank:** two sets of 5 lower and lifts each side

CORE E

- **Tabletop with Head Lift:** three sets of 15-second holds
- **Tabletop with Heel Touch:** two sets of 5 each leg
- ***Bridge on Ball with Lower and Lift:** three sets of 8
- **Leg Lift with Flat Band:** two sets of 10-second holds
- **Superman:** three sets of 10-second holds
- **Modified Side Plank:** two sets of 8 lower and lifts each side

CORE F

- **Tabletop with Heel Touch:** two sets of 7 each leg
- ***Full Plank:** two sets of 15-second holds
- ***Full Side Plank with Lower and Lift:** two sets of 15-second holds
- ***Frog:** two sets of 8
- ***Straight Leg Lower and Lift:** two sets of 5 each side

CORE G

- **Tabletop with Ball Squeeze:** three sets of 25-second holds
- **Tabletop with Heel Touch:** two sets of 8 each leg
- **Bridge on Ball with Lower and Lift:** three sets of 12
- **Leg Lift with Flat Band:** two sets of 15-second holds
- **Superman:** three sets of 20-second holds
- ***Side Plank:** two sets of 8 lower and lifts each side

CORE H

- **Full Plank:** two sets of 20-second holds
- **Full Side Plank with Lower and Lift:** two sets of 20-second holds
- **Frog:** two sets of 12
- **Straight Leg Lower and Lift:** two sets of 10 each side

CORE I

- **Tabletop with Ball Squeeze:** three sets of 30-second holds
- **Tabletop with Heel Touch:** two sets of 12 each leg
- **Bridge on Ball with Lower and Lift:** three sets of 15
- **Leg Lift with Flat Band:** two sets of 20-second holds
- **Superman:** three sets of 30-second holds
- **Side Plank:** two sets of 10 lower and lifts each side

CORE J

- **Full Plank:** two sets of 30-second holds
- **Full Side Plank with Lower and Lift:** two sets of 30-second holds
- **Frog:** three sets of 12
- **Straight Leg Lower and Lift:** three sets of 10 each side

ABDOMINAL COMPRESSION WITH LEG LIFT

Lie flat on your back, with a natural arch under your lower back. Bend your knees at a 90 degree angle and keep your heels on the floor and your toes pointed to the ceiling. As you exhale, lift your right foot off the floor, bringing your knee in line with your hip. Keep your shin parallel to the ceiling (maintain the 90 degree angle). Lift your head up off the floor and look at your knee. Hold for 10 inhales and exhales, then release. If you feel your neck straining, either lay your head back on the mat or support the back of your head with one hand.

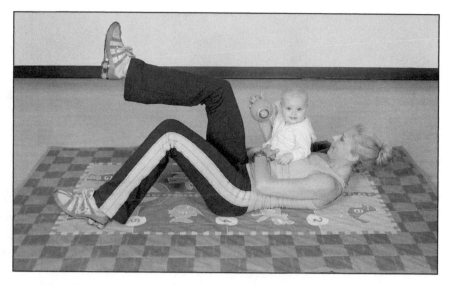

▲ ABDOMINAL COMPRESSION WITH LEG LIFT

BALL SQUEEZE BETWEEN ANKLES

Lie flat on your back with your knees bent and your arms extended out to the side for balance. Place a small ball between your feet and squeeze. Lift your feet off the floor and try to straighten your legs without locking your knee joint. The ability to straighten your legs will progress over time, so do not be surprised if they do not agree with being straight the first few times you perform this move. Tighten your quadriceps (thigh muscles) to help lengthen your hamstrings. Place pressure on the ball and hold for 10 seconds. Rest and repeat.

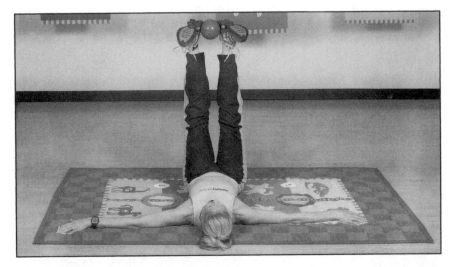

▲ BALL SQUEEZE BETWEEN ANKLES

BRIDGE

Lie flat on your back with your arms at your sides. Place your feet hip-distance apart, 8 to 12 inches from your glutes. Press into your feet, lifting your hips off the floor. Hold your hips up high, pulling your navel down. Don't forget to breathe! Hold for 15 seconds, and release back to the floor.

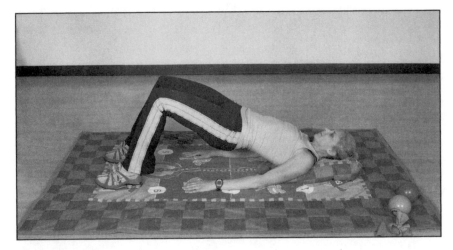

▲ BRIDGE

BRIDGE ON BALL WITH LOWER AND LIFT

Lie on the floor with a squeezable ball under the arch of your left foot and extend your right leg up (Figure 1). Keeping your right leg as straight as possible, press onto the ball and lift up your hips, creating a straight line from your knees to your shoulders with an exhale (Figure 2). Inhale as you lower, but do not touch the ground. Complete a set on the left side then move the ball to the other foot and repeat.

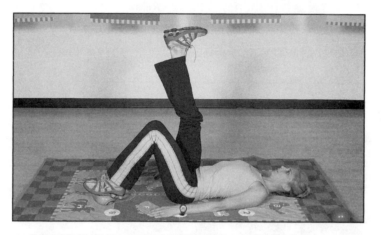

▲ BRIDGE ON BALL WITH LOWER AND LIFT, FIGURE 1

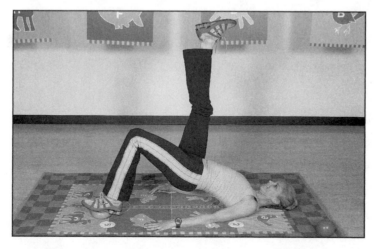

▲ BRIDGE ON BALL WITH LOWER AND LIFT, FIGURE 2

COMPRESSION

Lie flat on your back with your feet hip-distance apart, with your heels on the floor and your toes lifted. Pull your navel to your spine without flattening your back in to the mat. Check with one hand to make sure you are not pressing your low back into the floor; also, make sure you are not overarching your back. Breathe in through your nose and force the air out of your mouth 10 times. Repeat for 2 more sets of 10 breaths. This is a great move to do while entertaining your little one by counting to 10 in a foreign language or playing with a favorite toy. Be certain to maintain good form even if you're playing!

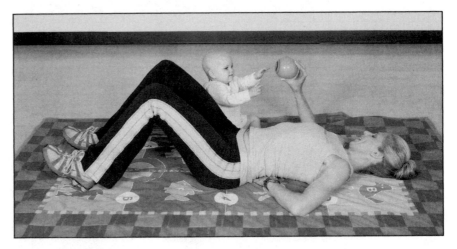

▲ COMPRESSION

FULL PLANK

Lie down and place your elbows on the floor, directly under your shoulders. Stretch your legs out behind you and lift up onto your elbows and your toes. Push back into your heels and keep your chin lifted. Hold for 15 seconds, rest for 30, and repeat a second time.

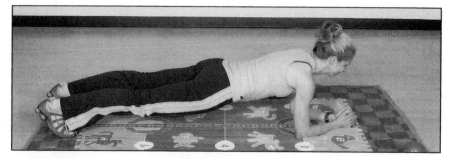

▲ FULL PLANK

FULL SIDE PLANK WITH LOWER AND LIFT

Lie on one side with your body in a straight line. Place your elbow on the floor directly under your shoulder. Stack your feet and lift your hips up off of the floor. Hold for 15 seconds, rest for 30, and repeat on this same side. Turn over and complete 2 sets on the other side of your body. While lifted, take a ball or toy and try to get the attention of your little one who should be an arm's reach from your body when performing this move!

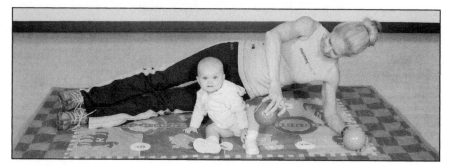

▲ FULL SIDE PLANK WITH LOWER AND LIFT

FROG

Begin by lying on your back, arms out, knees bent, holding a small squeezable ball between your heels (Figure 1). Exhale as you straighten your legs without locking the knees, and press your heels up toward the ceiling

(Figure 2). Release your legs slowly to the starting position and repeat 7 more times. Rest for 30 seconds and complete a second set.

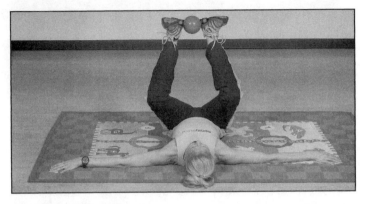

▲   FROG, FIGURE 1

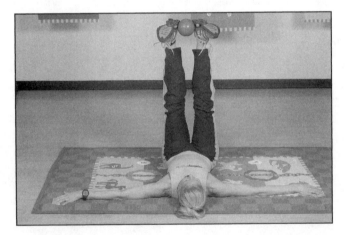

▲   FROG, FIGURE 2

LEG LIFT WITH FLAT BAND

Lying on your right side, tie a resistance tube or flat resistance band around your thighs just above your knee. Exhale as you lift your left leg up, hold for 10 seconds, then release. Repeat again on the same side before switching to the other side for 2 sets.

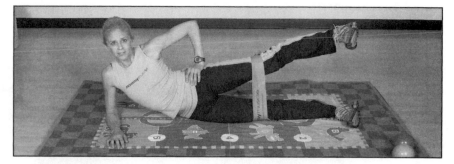

▲ **LEG LIFT WITH FLAT BAND**

MODIFIED PLANK

Lie on the floor. Place your knees and elbows on the floor with your elbows directly under your shoulders for good support. Keep your spine straight and your chin lifted as you lift your chest, stomach, and hips up off the floor (the only body parts left on the floor are your hands, forearms, elbows, knees, and toes). Do not allow your hips to pop up creating a V. Hold for 10 seconds, release, and repeat.

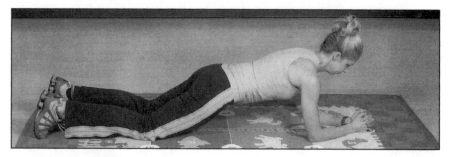

▲ **MODIFIED PLANK**

MODIFIED SIDE PLANK

Start by lying on your left side, with your body in a straight line. Bend at the knee, to a 90 degree angle. Make sure your elbow is directly under your shoulder. Lift your hips up off the ground with an exhale as you hold the position.

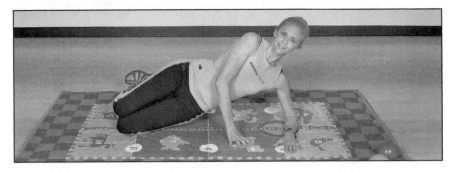

▲ MODIFIED SIDE PLANK

MODIFIED SIDE PLANK WITH LOWER AND LIFT

Start by lying on your left side, with your body in a straight line. Bend at the knee, to a 90 degree angle (Figure 1). Make sure your elbow is directly under your shoulder. Lift your hips up off the ground with an exhale, and then inhale as you release back toward the ground (Figure 2). Do not come all the way back to the floor. Make sure your elbow is under your shoulder for good support.

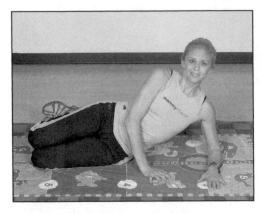

▲ MODIFIED SIDE PLANK WITH LOWER AND LIFT, FIGURE 1

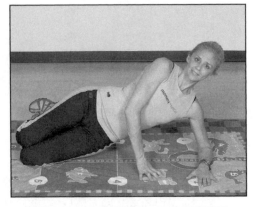

▲ MODIFIED SIDE PLANK WITH LOWER AND LIFT, FIGURE 2

SIDE PLANK

Start by lying on your left side, with your body in a straight line. Bend at the elbow. Make sure your elbow is directly under your shoulder. Lift your hips up off the ground and hold. Do not let your top shoulder come forward, even if placing your other hand on the floor to help steady you. Pull your navel back to your spine, and make sure you are breathing! Hold for 10 seconds, rest, and repeat. Then switch sides. If performing this move with your baby by your side, first make sure the baby is a safe distance from your body (the obliques are often weak after C-sections and pregnancy, and this exercise can be surprisingly difficult). For your sake and the baby's, place her a few feet away from your body. Grab a favorite toy and shake it gently, trying to pull her attention toward you and the toy. In a few weeks, you might even be able to sing a nursery rhyme to her while holding a side plank!

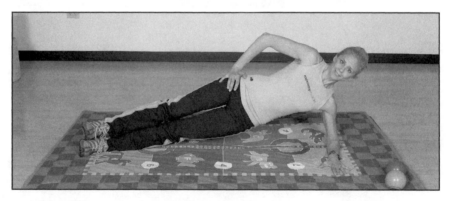

▲ SIDE PLANK

STRAIGHT LEG LOWER AND LIFT

Begin lying flat on your back with both feet up in the air (Figure 1). Holding your right leg in the starting position, lift your head as you lower your left leg toward the floor (Figure 2). Do not let your left leg touch the floor. Exhale as you bring your left leg back to the starting position. Complete 5 lower and lifts with the left leg, then switch to the right for 5 more.

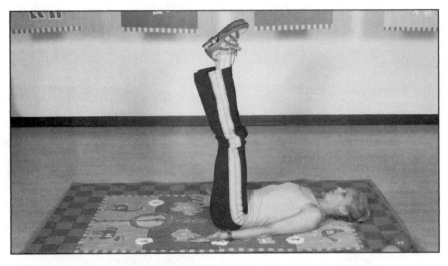

▲ STRAIGHT LEG LOWER AND LIFT, FIGURE 1

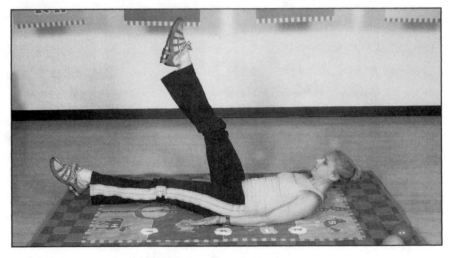

▲ STRAIGHT LEG LOWER AND LIFT, FIGURE 2

SUPERMAN

Come to an all-fours position on the floor. Extend your left arm out in front of you and your right leg back behind you. As you reach your fingertips and your toes away from each other, work to keep them in a nice straight line with no bend in the knee. Hold for 10 seconds and release, then repeat again before switching to the right arm and the left leg.

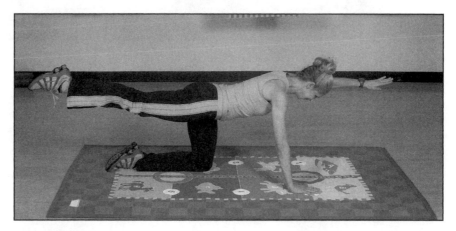

▲ SUPERMAN

TABLETOP WITH BALL SQUEEZE

Lie on the floor and place a small ball between your bent knees. Without arching your back, exhale and lift your feet up into tabletop position (knees in line with your hips and shins parallel to the ceiling). Hold for 10 inhales and exhales, release the feet back to the floor, rest, and then repeat. This exercise also allows for active play with your little one, or perhaps just a little extra side-by-side time.

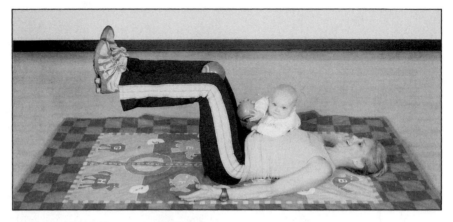

▲ TABLETOP WITH BALL SQUEEZE

TABLETOP WITH HEAD LIFT

Lie on the floor with your knees bent. Exhale and lift your feet up into tabletop position (knees in line with your hips and shins parallel to the ceiling), then lift your head up off the floor and hold for 15 seconds. Make a fist with your right hand and make sure your fist fits between your chin and your chest (this ensures proper position for the head and neck). If you feel strain in your neck, support your head with one hand.

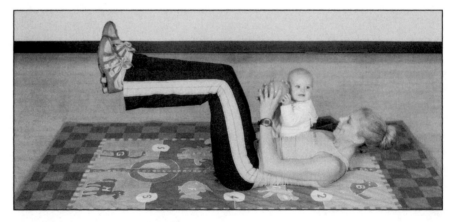

▲ TABLETOP WITH HEAD LIFT

TABLETOP WITH HEEL TOUCH

Begin in tabletop position with your head lifted. Hold your right leg still while dropping your left heel toward the floor with an inhale. Exhale as you return your left leg to tabletop position. Repeat 5 times, lowering your left leg, and then repeat 5 times, lowering your right leg. If your baby is by your side, take the opportunity to count in a foreign language for each repetition.

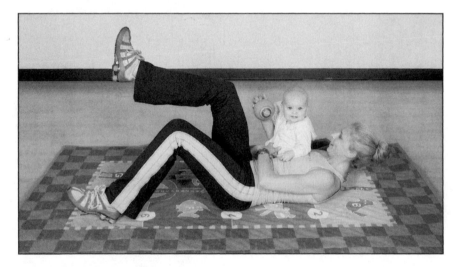

▲ TABLETOP WITH HEEL TOUCH

FULL BODY STRENGTH TRAINING

The Workouts

For these workouts, you will need a small squeezable ball (just a bit larger than a grapefruit) and a resistance tube. In the photos, I have used a figure 8 resistance tube as well as a standard resistance tube. Again, once the moves become too easy, add hand weights. Begin with 5-pound weights and increase them as necessary to 7, 8, 10, and then 12 pounds.

Since the body learns by repetition, you will be repeating the same exercises for four weeks at a time. If you get to the end of the set (10 to 12 repetitions of the same exercise) and you are not somewhat challenged by it, it is time to increase the repetitions you are doing in each set. You can add 2 to 3 repetitions to each move to gently challenge the body when need be. If the instruction is to hold a movement for 15 to 30 seconds and the time frame is not somewhat challenging, add 10 to 15 seconds to the move to signal to your body that it is time to grow stronger.

The ★ symbol before the name of an exercise is to inform you that this is a new exercise to be added onto the prior group of exercises.

FULL BODY WORKOUT A

- **Modified Push-up:** three sets of 12–15
- **Upright Rows:** three sets of 12–15
- **Rear Delt Fly:** three sets of 12–15
- **Biceps Curl:** three sets of 12–15
- **Triceps Dip:** three sets of 12–15
- **Pliéd Squat:** three sets of 12; add 3–5 lb weights in each hand
- **Stationary Lunge:** three sets of 12 each leg; add 3–5 lb weights in each hand
- **Calf Raise:** three sets of 12; add 3–5 lb weights in each hand
- **Glute Press:** three sets of 12 lower and lifts
- **Tabletop with Head Lift:** two sets of 15-second holds
- **Tabletop with Heel Touch:** two sets of 10 crunches
- **Tabletop Energize:** two sets of 5
- **Bridge on Ball with Lower and Lift:** three sets of 12
- **Superman:** two sets of 10: lower and lift in and out of pose
- **Modified Plank:** two sets of 10-second holds
- **Modified Side Plank:** two sets of 10 lower and lifts each side

FULL BODY WORKOUT B

- **Pliéd Squats:** three sets of 12–15 with 5–8 lb hand weights
- ***Forward Lunges:** three sets of 10 with 5–8 lb hand weights
- ***Single-Leg Bridge:** three sets of 5 each leg
- ***Push-ups with Ball under Hand:** three sets of 7 with ball under each hand
- **Upright Rows:** three sets of 12
- **Biceps Curl:** three sets of 12
- ***Triceps Extension:** three sets of 8 each side
- ***Rear Delt Row in V-Sit Position:** three sets of 8
- **Tabletop Energize:** two sets of 5 each side
- ***Full Plank:** two sets of 15-second holds

- ***Full Side Plank:** two sets of 15-second holds
- ***Frog:** two sets of 8
- ***Straight Leg Lower and Lift:** two sets of 5

FULL BODY WORKOUT C

- **Squats with Weights or Resistance Tubes:** three sets of 12
- **Lunges:** three sets of 12
- **Single-Leg Bridge:** three sets of 8 each leg
- **Push-ups with Ball under Hand:** three sets of 8 with ball under each hand
- **Upright Rows:** three sets of 12
- **Biceps Curl:** three sets of 12
- **Rear Delt Row in V-Sit Position:** three sets of 10
- **Triceps Extension:** three sets of 10 each side
- **Tabletop Energize:** two sets of 8 each side
- **Full Plank:** three sets of 20-second holds
- **Full Side Plank:** three sets of 20-second holds
- **Frog:** three sets of 10
- **Straight Leg Lower and Lift:** three sets of 5

FULL BODY WORKOUT D

- **Squats with weights or resistance tubes:** three sets of 15
- **Lunges:** three sets of 15
- **Single-Leg Bridge:** three sets of 10 each leg
- **Push-ups with Ball under Hand:** three sets of 10 with ball under each hand
- **Upright Rows:** three sets of 12
- **Biceps Curl:** three sets of 12
- **Rear Delt Row in V-Sit Position:** three sets of 12
- **Triceps Extension:** three sets of 12 each side
- **Tabletop Energize:** three sets of 8 each side
- ***Full Plank with Leg Lift:** three sets of 5-second holds on each side
- ***Full Side Plank with Lower and Lifts:** three sets of 8 on each side
- **Frog:** three sets of 12

- ***Straight Leg Lower and Lift, Both Legs:** three sets of 8

FULL BODY WORKOUT E

- ***1½ Pliéd Squats:** three sets of 8
- ***Reverse Lunges:** three sets of 10 each leg; add hand weights if necessary
- **Single-Leg Bridge:** three sets of 10 each leg
- ***Full Push-ups:** three sets of 8
- ***Shoulder Press in Lunge Position:** three sets of 8
- **Biceps Curl:** three sets of 15; increase the weights or shorten the resistance tube for more difficulty
- **Triceps Extension:** three sets of 15; increase the weights or shorten the resistance tube for more difficulty
- ***Cross N Reach:** three sets of 16 total crosses

FULL BODY WORKOUT F

- **1½ Pliéd Squats:** three sets of 10
- **Reverse Lunges:** three sets of 12 each leg; add hand weights if necessary
- **Single-Leg Bridge:** three sets of 12 each leg
- **Full Push-ups:** three sets of 12
- **Shoulder Press in Lunge Position:** three sets of 12
- **Biceps Curl:** three sets of 15; increase the weights or shorten the resistance tube for more difficulty
- **Triceps Extension:** three sets of 15; increase the weights or shorten the resistance tube for more difficulty
- **Cross N Reach:** three sets of 10 each side

FULL BODY WORKOUT G

- **1½ Pliéd Squats:** three sets of 15

- **Reverse Lunges:** three sets of 15 each leg; add hand weights if necessary
- **Single-Leg Bridge:** three sets of 15 each leg
- **Full Push-ups:** three sets of 15
- **Shoulder Press in Lunge Position:** three sets of 15
- **Biceps Curl:** three sets of 15; increase the weights or shorten the resistance tube for more difficulty
- **Triceps Extension:** three sets of 15; increase the weights or shorten the resistance tube for more difficulty
- **Cross N Reach:** three sets of 12 each side

FULL BODY WORKOUT H

- ***Jump Squats:** three sets of 10
- ***Walking Lunges:** three sets of 16 total lunges
- **Single-Leg Bridge:** three sets of 8 each leg
- ***Push-ups with Ball Transfer:** three sets of 10 transfers
- ***Upright Row, One-Legged Stance:** three sets of 10
- ***Overhead Pulldown:** three sets of 10
- **Biceps Curl:** three sets of 15
- ***Triceps Dip with Leg Extended:** three sets of 10
- ***Swim:** two sets of 16 total lift and lowers
- ***Full Plank with Rotation:** three sets of 6 each side
- ***Cross N Reach with Leg Lower and Lift:** three sets of 12 count (6 to each side, alternating sides)

FULL BODY WORKOUT I

- **Jump Squats:** three sets of 10
- **Walking Lunges:** three sets of 16 total lunges
- **Single-Leg Bridge:** three sets of 8 each leg
- **Push-ups with Ball Transfer:** three sets of 10 transfers
- **Upright Row, One-Legged Stance:** three sets of 10
- **Overhead Pulldown:** three sets of 10

- **Biceps Curl:** three sets of 15
- **Triceps Dip with Leg Extended:** three sets of 10
- **Swim:** two sets of 16 total lift and lowers
- **Full Plank with Rotation:** three sets of 6 each side
- **Cross N Reach with Leg Lower and Lift:** three sets of 12 count (6 to each side, alternating sides)

FULL BODY WORKOUT J

- **Jump Squats:** three sets of 12–15
- **Walking Lunges:** three sets of 24–30 total lunges
- **Single-Leg Bridge:** three sets of 12–15 each leg
- **Push-ups with Ball Transfer:** three sets of 12–18 transfers
- **Upright Row, One-Legged Stance:** three sets of 12–15
- **Overhead Pulldown:** three sets of 12–15
- **Biceps Curl:** three sets of 15
- **Triceps Dip with Leg Extended:** three sets of 15
- **Swim:** three sets of 16 total lift and lowers
- **Full Plank with Rotation:** three sets of 8 each side
- **Cross N Reach with Leg Lower and Lift:** three sets of 16 count (8 to each side, alternating sides)

1½ PLIED SQUATS

Begin in the pliéd squat start position (see page 108), then inhale and lower all the way down into the squat. As you exhale, come halfway back up, then lower back into the full squat, and exhale as you come back to the starting position. Repeat until completing 3 sets of 8 1½ squats. I always found the tempo of these squats matched up well with the song "Itsy Bitsy Spider." Why not perform these in front of your baby's high chair and entertain them with song while exercising?

CROSS N REACH

Begin flat on your back, and if your infant is able to hold his head steady and strong enough to sit up with little to no assistance, place him on your abdomen with his back against your legs, which extend up toward the ceiling. (Do not perform exercise with baby on belly unless you are certain that you can support him one-handed.) Take a ball in your left hand and reach the ball toward the outside of right leg, then release your upper body back to the floor. Perform 8 on the left side and 8 on the right. This exercise presents an opportunity for a fun game of peek-a-boo.

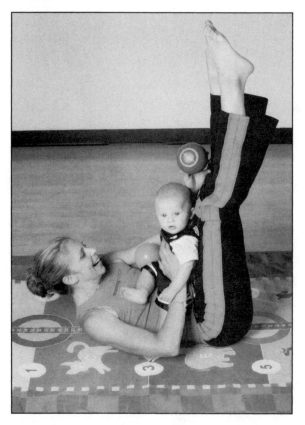

▲   CROSS N REACH

CROSS N REACH WITH LEG LOWER AND LIFT

Begin on your back with legs extended, as straight as they can be without locking your knees. Hold on to a small ball and have your arms extended overhead. Take the ball toward the outside of your right knee (your shoulders will lift off the floor) while dropping the left leg toward the floor. Release back to the starting position and reach the ball outside of your left leg, dropping the right toward the floor. Complete 2 sets of 12 (6 to each side, alternating sides).

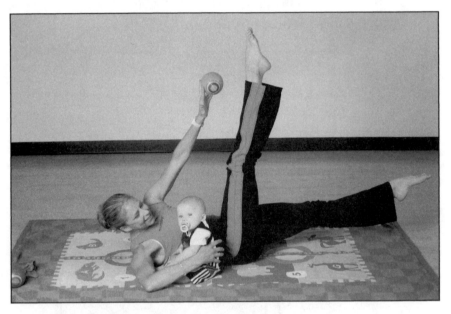

▲ CROSS N REACH WITH LEG LOWER AND LIFT

FORWARD LUNGES

Start in a standing position with your feet shoulder distance apart (Figure 1). Step your right foot out in front of you, and bend at the knee, dropping into a lunge (Figure 2). Press into your right foot as you return to a standing position. Repeat 10 times on your right side, and then switch to your left.

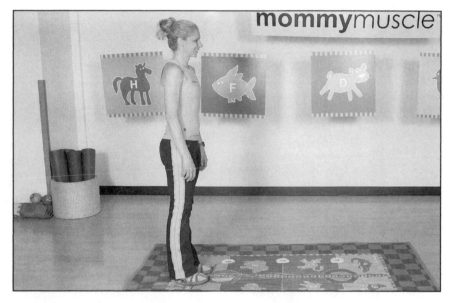

▲ FORWARD LUNGES, FIGURE 1

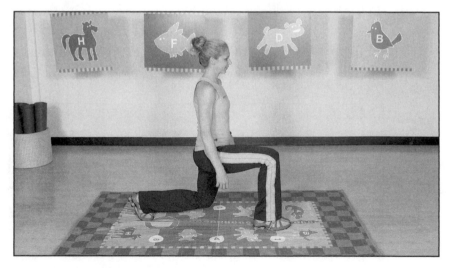

▲ FORWARD LUNGES, FIGURE 2

FULL PLANK WITH LEG LIFT

Begin in the full plank position. Lift your right foot up off the floor, straighten your leg, and hold for 5 seconds. Switch to the left leg and hold for 5 more seconds. Release out of the plank, resting on the floor before repeating for 2 more complete sets.

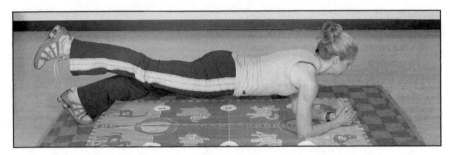

▲ FULL PLANK WITH LEG LIFT

FULL PLANK WITH ROTATION

Begin in the full side plank position (left side down; Figure 1). Reach your right hand underneath you and try to touch the floor with your fingertips on the inhale (Figure 2). Exhale as you twist the hips and shoulders back to the starting position. Repeat for a total of 6 repetitions before switching to the other side. Complete 2 full sets.

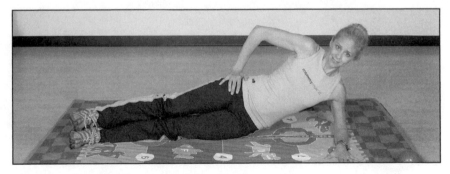

▲ FULL PLANK WITH ROTATION, FIGURE 1

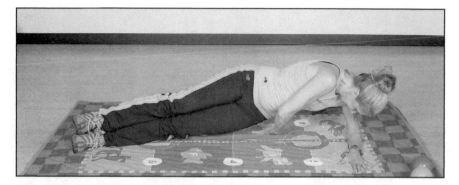

▲ FULL PLANK WITH ROTATION, FIGURE 2

FULL SIDE PLANK WITH LOWER AND LIFTS

Start in the full side plank position (Figure 1). On the inhale, release your hips down toward the floor, but not touching all the way (Figure 2). Exhale and press your hips back up until your body is in a straight line. Repeat 8 times on each side. Complete 2 sets of 8 on both sides of your body.

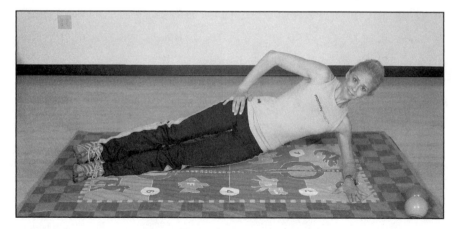

▲ FULL SIDE PLANK WITH LOWER AND LIFTS, FIGURE 1

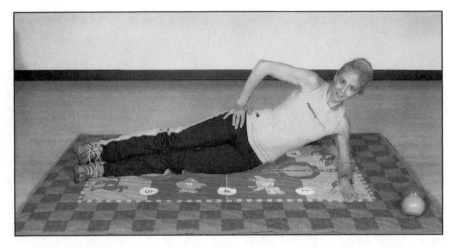

▲ FULL SIDE PLANK WITH LOWER AND LIFTS, FIGURE 2

FULL PUSH-UPS

Begin with your hands on the floor, wider than shoulder distance. Your arms and legs should be straight and legs are close together. You should be up on your toes, with your knees lifted off the floor. Gaze just out in front of you and inhale as you lower your body toward the floor by bending your elbows, exhale as you straighten the arms and press away from the floor back to the start position. Do 3 sets of 8.

JUMP SQUATS

Begin standing with your feet close together (Figure 1). Inhale as your bend the knees and jump your feet out wider than your shoulders (Figure 2), lowering into a squat position (Figure 3). Jump your feet back together as you return to the beginning position. Perform 3 sets of 8.

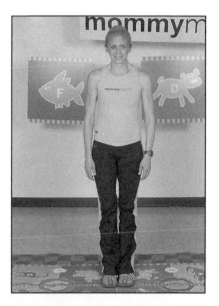

▲ JUMP SQUATS, FIGURE 1

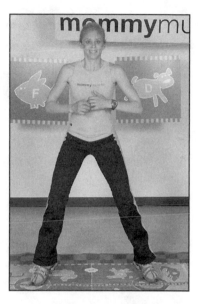

▲ JUMP SQUATS, FIGURE 2

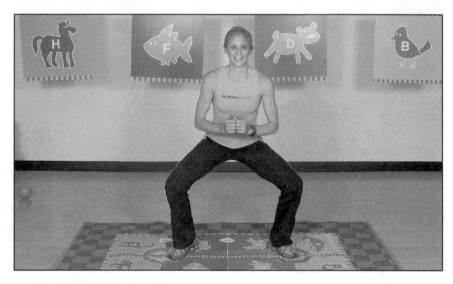

▲ JUMP SQUATS, FIGURE 3

UPRIGHT ROW, ONE-LEGGED STANCE

Place the resistance tube end under the arch of your left foot, and grab hold of the tube either by the handles or just below (for more resistance). Hinge forward slightly so that your right foot floats up off the floor (Figure 1). Exhale as you lift your hands up toward your collarbone (Figure 2) and then slowly release your hands back to the starting position while remaining balanced on the left foot. Perform 5 while balancing on your left foot and then an additional 5 while balanced on your right foot. Do 3 sets of 10.

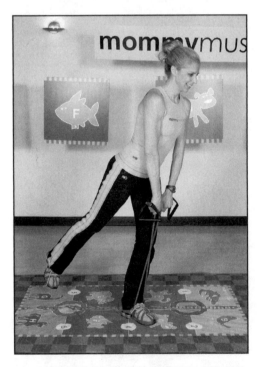

▲ UPRIGHT ROW, ONE-LEGGED STANCE, FIGURE 1

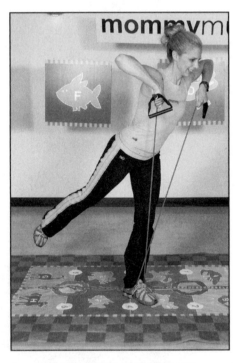

▲ UPRIGHT ROW, ONE-LEGGED STANCE, FIGURE 2

OVERHEAD PULLDOWN

Wrap the resistance tube around each hand and extend the arms overhead. Balance on the left leg and cross the right ankle over the left knee (if flexibility does not allow, just pick the foot up off the floor and hold it). (See Figure 1.) Pull your hands down toward your hips (Figure 2), keeping your arms straight (without locking your elbows), and then release your hands back overhead. Complete a set balancing on your left leg, the next on your right, and the final set balancing again on the left leg.

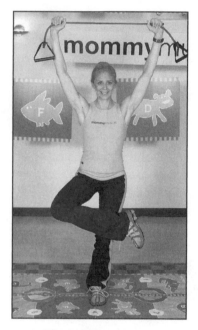

▲ OVERHEAD PULLDOWN,
FIGURE 1

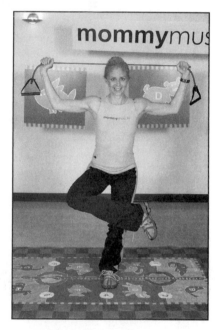

▲ OVERHEAD PULLDOWN,
FIGURE 2

PUSH-UPS WITH BALL TRANSFER

Begin in a push-up position (try the full push-up exercise on page 142 first) with a small ball under one hand (Figure 1). Bend your elbows and lower to the ground. After coming back to the starting position, roll the ball from one hand to the other (Figure 2) and perform another push-up. Complete 10 ball transfer push-ups, rest, and then complete 2 additional sets of 10. If the full push-up is too difficult, try this exercise in a mid-push-up form (Figure 3).

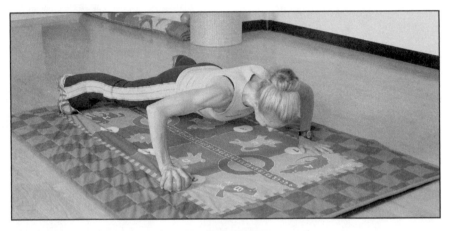

▲ PUSH-UPS WITH BALL TRANSFER, FIGURE 1

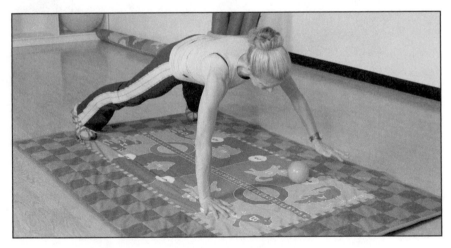

▲ PUSH-UPS WITH BALL TRANSFER, FIGURE 2

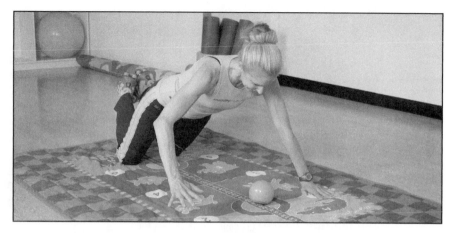

▲ PUSH-UPS WITH BALL TRANSFER, FIGURE 3

PUSH-UPS WITH BALL UNDER HAND

Begin on all fours, with your knees bent and your feet in the air. Place a small ball under your right hand (Figure 1). Lower down toward the floor. Exhale as you come back to the starting position. Complete 7 push-ups with the ball under your right hand, then put the ball under your left hand (Figure 2). Switch the ball from right to left 3 times for a total of 21 push-ups on each side.

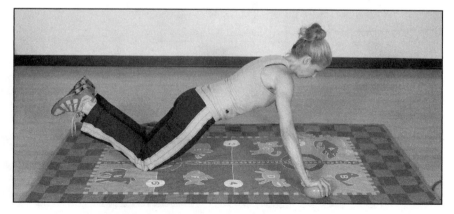

▲ PUSH-UPS WITH BALL UNDER HAND, FIGURE 1

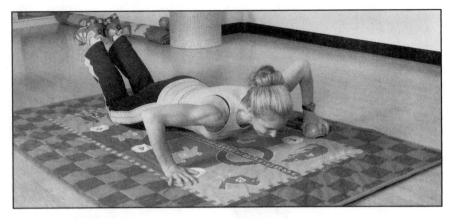

▲ PUSH-UPS WITH BALL UNDER HAND, FIGURE 2

REAR DELT ROW IN V-SIT POSITION

Start from a seated position on the floor, with your knees bent. Wrap the resistance tube around each of your feet one time. Hold a handle of the tube in each hand. Lean back so that your feet lift off the floor (Figure 1). Do not move your arms until you have found your balance. Exhale as you pull your elbows back, squeezing between your shoulder blades (Figure 2). Release slowly, repeating for a total of 8 times. Complete 3 sets of 8, bringing your feet to the floor in between sets.

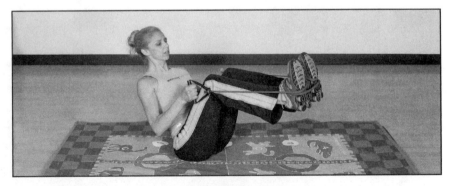

▲ REAR DELT ROW IN V-SIT POSITION, FIGURE 1

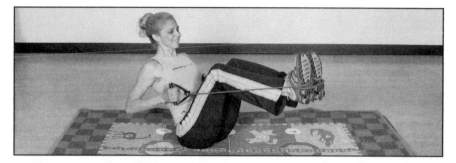

▲ REAR DELT ROW IN V-SIT POSITION, FIGURE 2

REVERSE LUNGES

You can add hand weights or an elastic band if you'd like to make this exercise more challenging (as shown in Figure 1). Begin in standing position with your feet hip-distance apart (Figure 1). Step your left leg back and lower into a lunge (Figure 2), then press off your front foot and return to standing. Take your right leg back into a lunge and then return to start. Continue alternating left and right legs for a total of 20 lunges. Rest and repeat for a total of 3 sets.

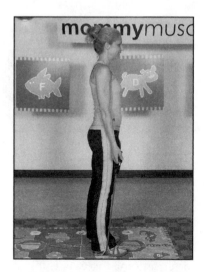

▲ REVERSE LUNGES, FIGURE 1

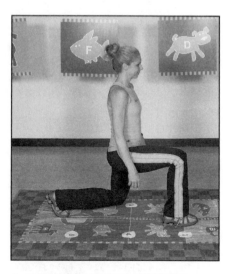

▲ REVERSE LUNGES, FIGURE 2

SHOULDER PRESS IN LUNGE POSITION

Begin in a stationary lunge position as shown, and place the resistance tube under the arch of your front foot. Holding the handles of the tube with your palms facing away from you, press your arms up overhead with an exhale, then release slowly back to the start position. Perform 4 overhead presses and then switch leg position, and complete another 4 presses. Rest and perform 2 more sets of 8 total presses.

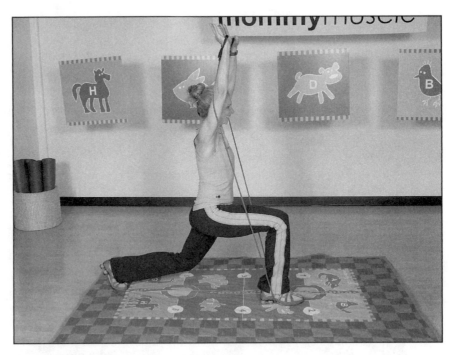

▲ SHOULDER PRESS IN LUNGE POSITION

SINGLE-LEG BRIDGE

Place a small ball under the arch of your left foot. Extend your right leg up. Inhale to prepare, exhale as you press your hips up to the ceiling. Lower down slowly; do not come all the way back to the floor.

Repeat 5 times on each side, 2 sets for a total of 10 repetitions each leg.

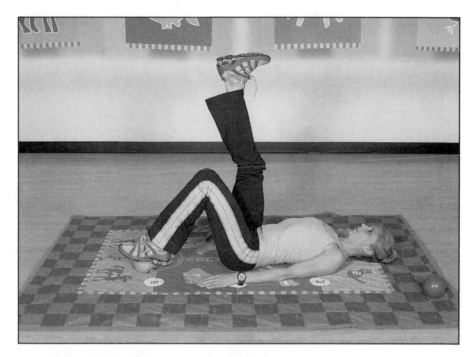

▲ SINGLE-LEG BRIDGE

STRAIGHT LEG LOWER AND LIFT, BOTH LEGS

Begin on your back with your arms by your sides, legs up toward the ceiling, and head flat on the floor (Figure 1). Lift your head as you lower your legs 4 to 6 inches closer to the ground (Figure 2). Exhale as you pull your legs back to the starting position. Repeat 8 times, rest, and then complete 2 more sets of 8.

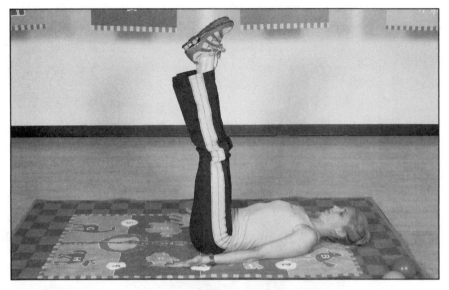

▲ STRAIGHT LEG LOWER AND LIFT, BOTH LEGS, FIGURE 1

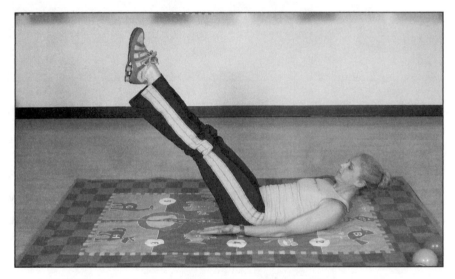

▲ STRAIGHT LEG LOWER AND LIFT, BOTH LEGS, FIGURE 2

SWIM

Lay down on your stomach with your arms and legs extended fully. Lift your right arm and left leg off the floor, then return them to the starting position. Next, lift your left arm and your right leg off the floor. Keep your arms and legs straight and find a rhythm to your breath that has you exhaling while lifting the right arm and left leg and inhaling on the alternate side. Complete 2 sets of 16. This exercise is a great time to play with your little ones. My babies loved to be right out in front of me and I would exhale like a strong wind during each move, causing them to squeal with delight!

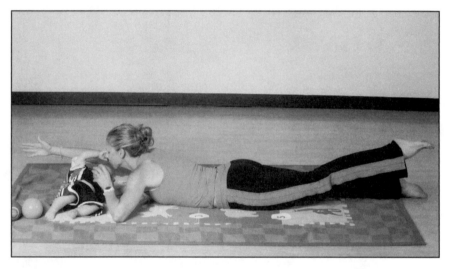

▲ SWIM

TABLETOP ENERGIZE

Begin in tabletop position with legs hip-distance apart with the small ball placed below your very lower back (Figure 1). Lower both feet toward the floor on an inhale (Figure 2). Exhale as you pull them back to tabletop. Only lower the legs as far as you can without changing the arch in your back. Remember to breathe, and do not hold on to the floor or mat!

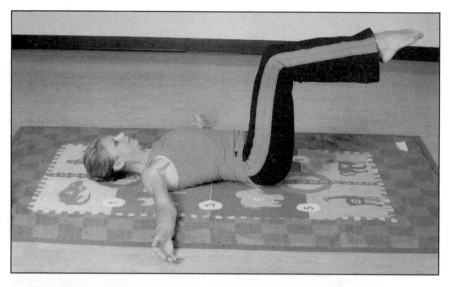

▲ TABLETOP ENERGIZE, FIGURE 1

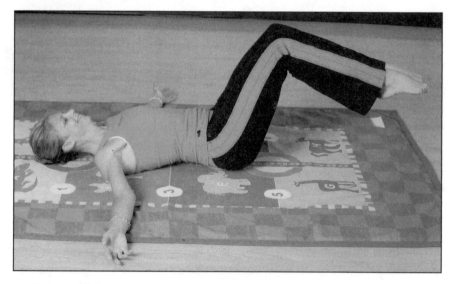

▲ TABLETOP ENERGIZE, FIGURE 2

TRICEPS DIP WITH LEG EXTENDED

Begin in the same position as you did for the triceps dip (Figure 1), then extend one leg out in front of you and keep it lifted off of the floor (Figure 2). Inhale as you bend your elbows, coming closer to the floor, and exhale as you straighten but do not lock your arms. Complete 3 sets of 10.

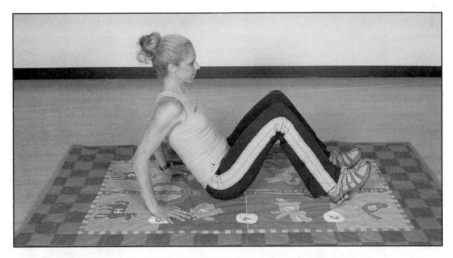

▲ TRICEPS DIP WITH LEG EXTENDED, FIGURE 1

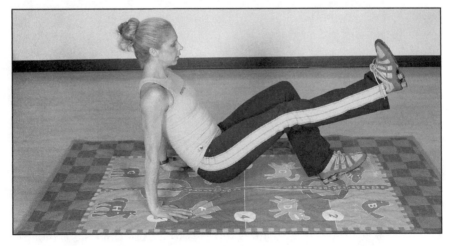

▲ TRICEPS DIP WITH LEG EXTENDED, FIGURE 2

TRICEPS EXTENSION

Stand with one foot slightly in front of the other. Hold one end (not the handle) of a resistance tube in each hand behind your back as shown in Figure 1. Inhale to prepare. On the exhale, extend your right arm up to the ceiling; do not lock your elbow (Figure 2). Release slowly. Complete 8 repetitions and then switch sides.

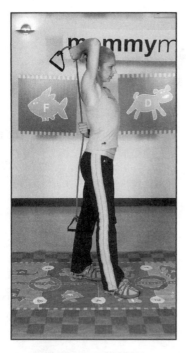

▲ TRICEPS EXTENSION, FIGURE 1

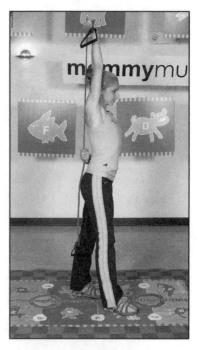

▲ TRICEPS EXTENSION, FIGURE 2

UPRIGHT ROWS

Stand on the resistance tube with your feet shoulder-length apart. You can cross the tube for more resistance if you like (Figure 1). Hold the handles of the tube so that your palms are facing your legs. Exhale as you pull your hands up toward your collarbone, keeping your upper arm and lower arm in line (Figure 2). Inhale as you release slowly.

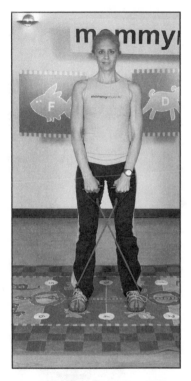

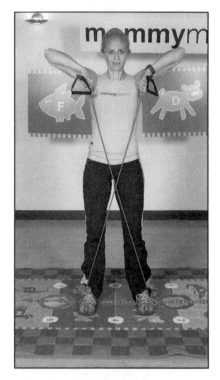

▲ UPRIGHT ROWS, FIGURE 1   ▲ UPRIGHT ROWS, FIGURE 2

WALKING LUNGES

These can be performed inside or outside and with the baby in a stroller or not! Take a large step forward with the right leg and lower into a lunge position. Exhale as you press up through the right heel, bringing the left foot forward and placing it on the ground next to the right foot. Then take your left foot forward and lower into a lunge, bringing the right foot forward to meet the left. Repeat for a total of 16 lunges in each of 3 sets.

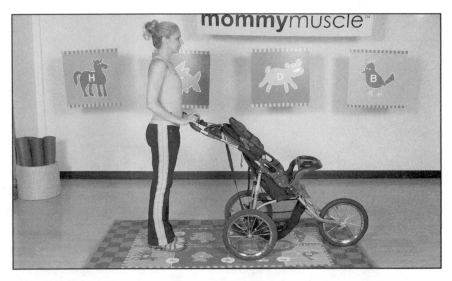

▲ WALKING LUNGES (WITH STROLLER), FIGURE 1

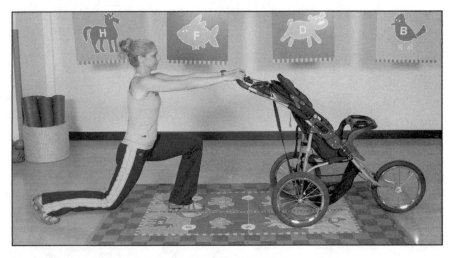

▲ WALKING LUNGES (WITH STROLLER), FIGURE 2

CARDIOVASCULAR CONDITIONING

Plan Ahead

For many new moms (yours truly included), getting off the baby weight is vital to feeling like we haven't been completely changed by motherhood. It can give you a sense of control over yourself and your life, and it can help you find balance and peace. Understanding how your body works at different effort levels is a must both for recovering from your delivery and meeting your goals in fitness, health, and clothing size!

Most moms don't have a lot of time to waste, and many barely have time to breathe, which is why having a plan and a strategy for each stage of recovery, fitness, and weight loss is important. It is also important to have a plan for each and every exercise session. This doesn't mean you have to have a *complicated* workout plan—it simply means having a goal of time and effort in mind and then following through. To properly plan for each workout, you must understand the energy systems of the body, what types of fuel they use, and how they feel when you use them. I have done much research on these topics and often had to read a book, chapter, or paper 10 times before I understood what they were saying! In hopes of you avoiding that, I have put the information into the simplest terms.

Your Heart Is a Muscle!

First off, it is important to remember that the heart is a muscle. Keeping the thought of the heart as a muscle can actually help us connect with the body and how aerobic conditioning strengthens the heart. Muscle tissues react to stress (exercise) by growing stronger, which means the muscle fibers knit themselves together more closely, taking up less space. This explains how you can build muscle and yet reduce your clothing size at the same time.

The same holds true for the heart muscle; the stronger it becomes from regular cardiovascular exercise such as walking, running, swimming, and cycling, the more compact the walls of the heart become. When this occurs, the heart actually has more interior space available for blood. This, in turn, allows more blood to enter the heart as it opens after each contraction. With more blood entering the heart, upon contraction, more blood leaves the heart. The end result is more oxygen and nutrients are delivered to each and every cell of the body with each and every beat of the heart, leading to the heart being called on to beat fewer times per minute. Less exertion from the heart with more energy delivery to the cells means less effort, less stress on your body, less energy expended due to fewer beats of the heart, and more energy available for other activities.

Effort Levels and Your Body's Fuel

Over time, the heart (as well as other organs and tissue) becomes increasingly efficient through regular exercise. For you, this means life becomes less and less fatiguing the more aerobically fit you become! Increased efficiency in the body is the result of the right level of effort during exercise. The higher your heart rate, the higher the level of exercise effort. You will need to determine your own exercise effort in one of three ways: perceived exertion, heart rate, or a combination of the two. I'll explain each of these ways in this chapter so you can figure out which one will work best for you. All three are good choices and are far better than not gauging or understanding your effort, which may leave you expending energy and time with little change.

The effort level you choose while exercising uses differing amounts of two types of fuel stored in your body. Think of it this way: Your body has two fuel tanks, a fat-storing one and one filled with carbohydrates. The carbohydrate gas tank is quite small and needs to be refilled any and every time it is used. The fat gas tank (this is not a reflection on a person's size—from skinny to not skinny, the same holds true) has unlimited resources and is much larger than the carbohydrate tank. In fact, the fat tank has nearly endless amounts of energy in it. When you expend fuel from your carbohydrate tank and don't replace it right away, you can begin to suffer from fatigue, food cravings, muscle cramps, and moodiness; you will continue to feel this way until the gas tank has been refilled. When you pull energy from your fat tank, your body hardly notices because it has a seemingly endless supply. As a matter of fact, oftentimes the more fat you burn, the better you feel!

The higher your heart rate (effort), the more carbohydrates the body is forced to use. During some levels of exercise effort, there is hardly any, if any at all, fat being used. Many of us have heard for decades that the harder the effort, the better. This is true if you want to be sore, tired, cranky, and storing fat. If those are not your goals, participate in exercise at a moderate effort, conserving carbohydrates and expending fat, which will leave you more energetic after the exercise than before and perhaps even during.

Gauging Your Effort Through Heart Rate

You can also determine how hard your body is working by calculating your heart rate. To assess your effort by heart rate alone, you must own a heart rate monitor so that the number of times your heart is beating per minute is displayed on a wristwatch. The number you see then needs to be translated into a percentage of the highest heart rate your body is capable of producing (maximal heart rate). For instance, my maximal heart rate is 179 beats per minute. If I wanted to exercise at a level of 65 percent in hopes of speeding recovery and maximizing fat burning, I would then try to maintain a heart rate of 117 beats per minute. The following would be my personal heart rate numbers and percentages for each of the training zones described above.

Active Recovery
65 percent—117 BPM (beats per minute)
Endurance (Fat Burning)
70 percent—126 BPM
75 percent—135 BPM
80 percent—143 BPM
Threshold Training
85 percent—153 BPM
90 percent—161 BPM
Anaerobic/VO2 Max Efforts
92 percent—165 BPM

Your maximal heart rate can be determined by a simple mathematical equation. (Although this is scientifically based, it is still an estimate and your true numbers can only be known through a VO2 max test, which can be costly and still has a margin of error.) Many universities offer this test and some fitness facilities do as well. (For a list of fitness facilities, visit *www.newleaffitness.com*.) For a good estimate of your maximal heart rate, take the number 220 and deduct from it your current age.

When you first begin to gauge your effort through use of a heart rate monitor, you may want to carry with you a note card with your intended heart rate numbers and zones on it as a reminder of the right effort to be in.

Buying a Heart Monitor

While many heart rate monitors have lots of bells and whistles, and complicated programs that come along with them, the following are a few functions you should look for in a monitor.

- **Stopwatch**
- **Alarm functions:** This will allow you to set your lowest desired heart rate for exercise as well as your highest desired number. The watch will then beep at you if you sink below your bottom number or go above your highest number, helping you to maintain the desired heart rate and reach your goal.
- **Time of day:** Moms are always on such tight schedules, and this function is a nice one to have.
- **Weekly summary of minutes exercised:** The numbers don't lie! Sometimes we think we have done more than we actually have, and there is no way to get the results without putting in the time!

One function that exercisers often love but that can do them more harm than good when it comes to weight loss is that of total calories burned during exercise. This function delivers an estimate—scientifically based, yes—but still an estimate. And while it may be based on your age, sex, height, and weight, the monitor does not know your body composition nor your efficiency level, both of which play a major role in how many calories you burn per minute during exercise. The number displayed on the monitor in this function represents the total calories burned, including both fat calories and carbohydrate calories. More often than not, this can lead to overeating postexercise!

I myself am guilty of looking at this number after exercise and thinking "*Wow*, I can eat whatever I want now! I just burned 500 calories." However, there's much more to the story.

The Real Truth Behind the "Calories Burned" Estimate

When looking at this number, remember that we can burn a whole bunch of fat calories, and our bodies don't mind at all. In fact, they want you to give away fat, and that means you do not need to replenish them. You do, however, want to replace the carbohydrate calories that were expended during exercise so that you can maintain your energy and not crash and burn. My practice and belief is that the carbohydrate calories should be replenished, but not the fat!

I recommend using the following chart★ as an estimate of the percentage of fat and carbohydrates burned at varying levels of intensity.

PERCENTAGE OF FAT AND CARBOHYDRATES BURNED AT VARYING LEVELS OF INTENSITY				
65% Effort	70–80% Effort	85% Effort	90% Effort	92% Effort
60% fat	50% fat	30% fat	10–20% fat	0% fat
40% carb	50% carb	70% carb	80–90% carb	100% carb

★ *This chart is an estimate and is based on the results of hundreds of VO2 max tests that I have performed over four years' time. The numbers are generalities meant to give you an idea of energy usage and may not apply to all individuals. For percentage and numbers that apply directly to you, either have a VO2 max test done or work with a registered dietitian/ licensed nutritionist as well as an exercise physiologist to determine more precise/personal numbers and percentages.*

If you really want to figure out how many calories you burned, get the total calories burned estimate from your monitor, find your average heart rate for the workout (this should be stored in the watch), and divide that total number by the percentage of carbohydrate use estimated in the chart above for that heart rate.

So if your heart rate monitor assumes you burned 350 calories while at an average of 75 percent effort, you will complete the following equation:

350 x 50% = 175 carbohydrate calories burned and in need of replenishment

It is best to replenish the expended carbohydrate calories within 30 to 45 minutes postexercise to avoid a dip in energy. Because losing weight is only achieved if you take in fewer calories than you burn every day, if you replenished all 350 calories expended in the exercise example above, then the effort was all for naught when it comes to weight loss. Yes, fitness can be accumulated from each and every exercise effort, even those where all calories expended are replenished, but weight loss and fitness may both be achieved if you keep a close eye on how much replenishment your body actually needs.

Exercise Efforts/Training Zones/Perceive Exertion

Exercise efforts are typically broken down into the following zones:

- Recovery
- Aerobic Conditioning (Endurance/Fat Burning)
- Threshold (Lactate) Training
- Anaerobic Conditioning (Maximal Oxygen Uptake, or VO2 Max Efforts)

Each zone is defined by how hard your heart is working during the exercise session. Along with an explanation of the zones, you'll find descriptions of how each zone feels when you are in it. These feelings are called perceived exertion and are important measures of what training zone and fuel source you are using.

The Recovery Zone

The recovery effort is actually "active recovery," which means moving at a gentle pace that takes place at or around 65 percent of your maximum heart rate. This effort flushes stress, increases oxygen delivery and use, speeds nutrients to every cell of the body, and does not drain your energy resources as it uses mostly fat for fuel. This type of effort can be thought of as a healer and as a pick-me-up, and it could be performed every day; it has no ill effects on the body. At this effort, you are able to move with good form, which translates to proper muscle usage and a low risk of injury. While in the recovery zone (again, at 65 percent effort), you will usually notice the following:

- A slight increase in breathing, but still fully controlled breathing
- A light sweat
- A slight increase in body temperature, just enough to feel warmth or heat below the skin
- Feelings of relief, confidence, and happiness
- Stimulation of the body and mind; feeling awake and energetic

In the first few weeks, perhaps months, after a C-section, the recovery zone is a great place to exercise, as it will speed the healing process. However, you must at some point increase your efforts so that we increase your fitness level. While the recovery zone has many benefits, such as reducing stress, increasing the blood flow, and moving more oxygen and nutrients to the body, it typically does not increase your fitness level. But increasing your fitness level makes the rest of your life less fatiguing and easier. Be patient and stay in this zone to begin with, but also make a mental note to yourself that soon this will not be effort enough.

This zone is perfect when life becomes too much to handle and you feel you are at the end of your rope physically, mentally, and emotionally. It can help to alleviate such feelings without adding to them! When your energy levels are zip, exercise in this zone and tell yourself that something is always better than nothing.

The Aerobic Conditioning Zone

The aerobic conditioning zone or effort level usually takes place between 70 and 80 percent of your maximal heart rate. While it can possibly mean up to 10 additional beats of the heart per minute, it is generally thought of as a low-stress, moderate effort workout. It is still placing stress on the body, but the level is low enough that the body does not need a day or two to recover from it, yet it is just hard enough that it signals the body to become more fit and use oxygen more efficiently.

This effort is often referred to as a "fat burning" effort and rightfully so. Not only does it typically burn more fat calories than easier and harder efforts, but also the more time you spend at this effort, the better you become at using oxygen, which aids in the breakdown of fat for fuel. Thus, the more you practice this effort, the better you become at breaking down and using fat for fuel. While performing at this effort, the body, the mind, and the spirit might notice the following:

- Feelings of confidence, strength, and energy
- Noticeable effort, noticeable work at a level that does not have the brain questioning the body's ability

- The ability to say your entire name without gasping for air
- Controlled form and breath (no heavy or rapid breathing)
- A noticeable rise in body heat, and moderate sweating
- A sense of balance, that every request for oxygen and energy that the working muscles generate is easily met
- Sustainability; even though you are working, it is an effort that you could sustain for at least 30 minutes
- Absence of discomfort, no pain or burning beneath the skin

The aerobic zone is the zone where the body stands to gain the most fitness. It is just enough of a challenge to encourage growth in the body, and due to the fact that it does not disturb the body's balance, you are capable of performing this effort daily. You should need no recovery time between efforts as long as you give your body proper calorie intake, fluid intake, and sleep. For many new moms, it is difficult to maintain balance in the body due to the physically demanding nature of motherhood. Therefore, even though your body possesses the ability to exercise daily, doctors do not recommended that brand-new moms participate in cardiovascular conditioning daily. And it is recommended that a day (or days) of complete rest (absence of exercise) be part of your routine as well. As a matter of fact, rest should always be a part of your exercise plan. Plan a day without exercise into every week. Three months after you have begun to exercise, you can increase your cardio efforts to five days per week if you feel you have the energy, time, and need to boost the weight loss process a bit. However, for most moms, four days will be sufficient.

Threshold (Lactic Acid) Efforts

There is a point at which exercise efforts disturb the balance in the body. Once exertion levels become high enough, typically around 85 percent of your maximal capacity, the body begins using more carbohydrates and less fat for fuel. The body breaks down the carbohydrates, uses the fuel, and leaves behind pyruvic acid. Pyruvic acid is further broken down, leaving lactic acid behind. When the exercise level is moderate, the body can sweep lactic acid away before it accumulates. In higher heart rates, and at threshold efforts, the body cannot flush the lactic acid quickly enough, and its accumulation causes discomfort in the form of a burning sensation. The buildup of lactic acid also begins to interfere with the messages being sent back and forth between the brain and the body. This communication breakdown leads to bad form and increases the risk of injury to the body. Not only does a burning sensation begin to increase, but your rate of respiration also increases, and your lungs work harder to expel the carbon dioxide that is released into the body (as carbohydrates and oxygen are used at a higher rate for the harder effort). The following are symptoms and feelings typical of exercise at the threshold level:

- A burning sensation in your muscles
- A fast-paced breath, and loss of control over breath
- Feelings of weakness
- Separation of the brain and the body; they are no longer in harmony, and the brain will often begin to tell you to slow down, back off, or stop the effort all together
- Increased body temperature, oftentimes to a seemingly unbearable level
- Increased perspiration
- Increased desire to stop
- Feelings and thoughts of not being able to sustain the effort for much longer
- A general dislike for the effort

Because the body is out of balance at this effort, it takes significant mental fortitude to continue at this level. It is also possible for participants to actually feel more energetic during this effort and often experience what is called a "runner's high." It is vital that you realize these feelings of energy and elation are temporary—very temporary—and that the high you feel will soon be replaced with a very big decline in energy due to an excessive use of carbohydrates at this effort and little fat burning.

More often than not, exercisers who repeat this effort find themselves unable to control their food intake and experience many food cravings. Expending too many carbohydrate calories during exercise can place the body in a carbohydrate deficit. With carbohydrates being the only type of fuel that feeds the brain, which controls the whole body, you simply cannot live without them. If you continue to operate in a deficit, sooner or later you will give in to the cravings and find yourself consuming more calories than you body actually needs. Continuing to exercise at this effort can lead to what I call the carbohydrate merry-go-round, during which exercisers are gaining and losing the same few pounds over and over again, making little sustainable change in the body and becoming increasingly frustrated with the lack of change.

Since carbohydrates are stored in the body by binding to water, when you use the carbohydrates for exercise, you shed the water. Many exercisers can store a few pounds worth of this water/carbohydrate mixture known as glycogen, and after three to four difficult exercise sessions may find themselves two or three pounds lighter. Feeling successful, they continue to exercise at the threshold level until they are too fatigued to continue. During the next few days while the exercisers rest, the foods eaten will be stored in the body, restoring the levels of glycogen. After a few days, the exercisers will find themselves having added back on those two to three pounds, and frustration sets in. Oftentimes this frustration and lack of sustainable change lead to a belief that exercise is just a waste of time and is not helping. Sooner or later, many find themselves burned out, and they may discontinue participation in the activities they had hoped would help change their fitness levels and body compositions.

Because of the intense effort, many exercisers feel they are gaining more fitness at the threshold level than at levels not quite so intense. Again, the results are short term and will only be sustained as long as the exerciser is able to continue working out at this effort. I have found that many exercisers cannot sustain this level of intensity for more than three to four months before burnout or injury occurs. Many times, I have also witnessed a negative body composition change from this effort, which means the exercisers notice initial weight loss but then begin to gain the weight back and often end up heavier than when they began their exercise program. For a new mom, I do not recommend this effort level, not only because of the energy expenditure and risk of injury but also because it can cause an emotional rollercoaster. Higher heart efforts such as threshold training raise the levels of cortisol (stress hormone) found in the body, leaving the exerciser more stressed out, less confident, and at a higher risk of depression, none of which are optimal for anyone, but especially a sleep-deprived, over-exerted new mom!

Threshold training efforts at or around 85 percent of maximal effort are necessary for those seeking increased athletic performance. But for the rest of us, it should be a place we avoid, a signal that we are over-stressing our bodies and decreasing the levels of carbohydrates available in the body instead of decreasing the fat!

Anaerobic (VO2 Max) Efforts

While many do experience a high and feel that threshold training makes them more fit, it is actually too hard to recover from daily. Though it does induce stress, it is actually not enough stress or effort to increase our VO2 max (the amount of oxygen a person takes in and puts to use). The effort level necessary for VO2 max increase typically occurs at 92 percent of our maximal capacity. At such an intensity, the body utilizes the fast-twitch muscle fibers for movement, which do not use oxygen or burn fat. This effort not only uses carbohydrates solely for movement but also uses them at such a high rate that the body requires up to 72 hours of recovery before it could be ready to repeat the effort.

With the increase in heart rate comes an increase in the release of toxins and cortisol as well as a decrease in serotonin, the "happy hormone." Participation in this effort requires constant attention to form, planned recovery, and typically a daily increase in carbohydrates. You should expect fatigue and muscular soreness from these efforts for up to 48 hours postexercise. Participants will also notice the following signs and symptoms during exercise:

- A very rapid rate of respiration and gasping of air
- An increased rate of perspiration
- A deep burning sensation in the legs and perhaps the lungs
- An increased sense of losing control
- An increased feeling of fatigue and weakness
- A decreased feeling of strength and fortitude
- An increased desire to slow down or stop exercise
- A possible loss of good form and posture
- A decrease in the time that the effort can be sustained (typically not more than 30 seconds)

Participating in efforts at 92 percent of maximal capacity is often done in interval training sessions, where the participant will work hard for a period of time, achieving the desired heart rate in the last 30 seconds of the effort, then participate in active recovery (65 percent effort) for an equal amount of time before returning to the harder effort again. Such types of interval maximal efforts should only be done as long as good form is maintained and not more than one effort per week. Trainers also recommend that interval training at this level only take place during the eight weeks leading up to an athletic event and then be discontinued for a period of time following the event. Because of the high cost to the body and the high risk of injury, I rarely recommend this level of training for anyone who is looking to increase their overall health and well-being, and especially not for those looking to achieve fat loss through exercise.

Which Zone Is Right for You?

It really boils down to this: The higher the heart rate, the more carbohydrates (energy) you are expending and the less fat you are burning. Since carbohydrates are not an energy source that your body likes to run low on or out of (and since your body does not perform well when it is low or out of carbohydrates), it is vital to motherhood that you do not overexpend carbohydrates during exercise. Expending fat during exercise not only ensures that you maintain energy for motherhood and all it brings daily, but also can lower your risk of disease and other medical conditions that could negatively affect your health and the well-being of your families. Is it important that you memorize all of the above zones? No—but it is vital to your well-being that you understand the "cost" to the body when the proper exertion level is not achieved or overachieved.

The bottom line is that the more moderate exercise efforts are best for new moms. They reduce the risk of knee and hip injury, which new moms are at higher risk for. In Chapter 4, I discussed the postural changes that occur in pregnancy—I often refer to them as "structural damage." Yes, the damage is temporary, if you work to restructure the body through proper strength and core training. But until that structure is properly stabilized, your knees and hips are at risk of injury. So for those of us anxious to return to our old selves, again think about the fact that too much too soon brings with it the potential for injury. It is far better, in my opinion, to slowly work your way back and be able to exercise regularly than to dive in, end up injured, and then be forced to forgo exercise for six to twelve weeks while the proper healing process takes place. The results will come much sooner if you can participate daily in moderate activity for three to four months in a row versus working out hard for one month and then hitting the couch hard for the next two months.

MOM TO MOM: LOSING 50 POUNDS . . . THREE TIMES!

The first time I set out to lose 50 pounds was not due to weight gain during pregnancy. It was due to 15 years of smoking, lack of exercise, eating fast food, and a general lack of knowledge or desire for good health. I began an exercise program and diet and the 50 pounds came off over a year's time. Looking back, I wish I had understood how hard or not hard to work out! My workouts were so doggone hard, and they didn't have to be. Actually, had they been a little easier, I would no doubt have ended up at my goal weight a few months earlier. I truly believed back then that the harder the workout was, the faster I would lose the weight and the better I would feel. Wrong! Harder is better is a very easy trap to fall into.

When I went to lose 50 pounds the second two times, after my babies were born, I exercised a lot smarter. Although I owned a heart rate monitor, I found it too depressing to use! All it did was remind me of how fit I used to be and how unfit I had become, so I banished the monitor and found ways of measuring my effort without it. My clues were this . . . if I could not say my full name without gasping for air, then I was working too hard and needed to ease up. If I was able to belt out a show tune or "God Bless America," then my effort wasn't hard enough. But if I could say three or four words without gasping, then I was on track. Another system I used to measure exertion is the chewing gum test. For this form of measurement, if I am working at too low of an effort, I will be able to blow a bubble; if I am exercising at too high of a level, I will feel the need to spit out the gum. But if I am exercising at the right level, I can hold the gum in my mouth without it being bothersome! These assessments of effort may not work for everyone. They are reflective of the signals that my body gives to me, and they are also reflective of what my number one goal has been—weight loss/weight management, better health, and good energy. ~Mary Beth

Combining Heart Rate, Perceived Exertion, and Training Zones

I feel the best results come from wearing a heart rate monitor as well as gauging effort by how your body feels. Our bodies are never the same two days in a row: Fatigue, energy levels, hours of sleep, hydration levels, stress, hormones, and challenges to the immune system fluctuate daily. The result of these fluctuations is that one day, 75 percent exercise effort feels moderate, and the next day it can feel horribly difficult.

Forcing yourself to stay at 75 percent when it feels awful is like adding insult to injury. You already have so many demands on your life as a mom that forcing an effort when your body just doesn't have it to give that day will not only deny you the physical benefits of the effort, but it can also mess with your emotional stability (with thoughts such as "I feel horrible today, what is wrong? Why am I so out of shape? I will never be the same.") as well. It is for this reason that matching the number with the heart rate will give you the best form of guidance.

Listen to your body, and when your effort level feels much higher than the percentage of effort you are seeing on the watch, back off. Nine times out of ten when my effort feels extreme and the heart rate monitor does not reflect the effort, I usually begin showing signs of a cold within the next few days, or I finally admit how exhausted I am and allow myself a morning of sleeping in or a long nap on a weekend afternoon. After the rest that my body has signaled me to take, I am always right back to feeling the way I like and seeing the numbers reflected accurately on my heart rate monitor.

Take this guidance and listen to your body, and it will respond, it will change, and it will become your friend again.

Take Your Time

It generally takes eight weeks to build a solid aerobic fitness base. Given the major surgery, major changes in your posture, and major change on your available time, you should take 12 weeks to get there. This is not because you can't do it in eight; it is because things will come up that require you to push a workout or three off to the side each week. You won't mind rearranging your schedule—after all, the schedule changes are usually due to that little angel asleep down the hall. Patience is a gift, and giving yourself a few extra weeks to build this base will only help you in the long run. Forcing it when life gets in the way won't help at all, but neither will dragging it out until your baby's first birthday.

It is very possible that by the end of month three, you will find yourself having to walk much faster or perhaps choose a route that has many hills in an effort to keep your heart rate at 75 percent. If this is the case, you might want to begin intervals of running and walking to achieve the intended heart rate. However, *do not run at all until at least eight weeks post-C-section*. Keep in mind that the hormone relaxin is still in your system and is affecting your tendons and ligaments. You also may want to incorporate this routine into just one or two of your cardio efforts per week, and if your effort while running climbs higher than 75 percent, slow down or ease back into a walk.

MOM to MOM: DOING TOO MUCH TOO SOON

Hindsight is for sure 20/20. While I was pregnant with my first baby, I kept hearing from other moms how they hadn't lost all their baby weight and I was determined not to be one of them. I love to be active and can't sit still, so I began exercising almost immediately. I took my son, Colin, for a walk the day we were home from the hospital, and two days later I was on a speedwalk while I was waiting for my midwife to call me back and give me the OK to work out. By 10 days I was on the elliptical, and by four weeks I was trying to run. I say "try" because running was causing me a lot of pain. But I pressed through, trying over and over. Running is such a great way to burn calories, and it gives me such a great adrenaline release. I also just wanted to prove that I could get back to the shape I was before the baby, including running as fast, and as long—not just fitting into my clothes.

I did end up losing all of the weight and fitting into my prepregnancy clothes by the time my son was 12 weeks old, but I had to give up running for several months. As it turns out, my body needed more time to recover before I could get back into running. I experienced a number of joint issues and was often really sore and fatigued. I finally stopped running for a few months to allow my body to heal and progress at a safe, slower pace. Not only did my body feel better, but my energy levels increased as well.

Fast forward two years and another baby boy! This time I am taking a different approach. I haven't even attempted running, and won't for another few weeks, until I am 16 to 18 weeks postpartum. I still have a few pounds, and a jean size to go, but I know I will get there soon. My approach today is slower, but steady. I work daily to improve my health and fitness but not at the expense of my body or my energy! I no longer feel like I have something to prove. I have learned that listening to my own body is the most important thing, that making an effort is vital, but not expecting overnight results is also vital. ~Danielle

How to Transition from Walking to Running

If you have gained enough fitness that your heart rate is remaining low while walking, to get a heart rate of 75 percent or beyond, you will have to start running. However, most of us can't just start running for 30 minutes straight without our heart rates going way up! This plan will help you make a smooth transition from walking to running. It's very important to progress safely and slowly, so take it one week at a time as you increase your effort. As you can see, it can easily take three months to accomplish this goal. Whenever you find yourself at this point in your training—needing to work harder to increase your heart rate—implement this twelve-week transition plan from walking to running.

First Transition Week

- Walk 5 minutes to warm up
- Run 1 minute, walk 4 minutes (Repeat 5 times)
- Walk 5 minutes to cool down

Second Transition Week

- Walk 5 minutes to warm up
- Run 2 minutes, walk 3 minutes (Repeat 5 times)
- Walk 5 minutes to cool down

Third Transition Week

- Walk 5 minutes to warm up
- Run 4 minutes, walk 1 minute (Repeat 5 times)
- Walk 5 minutes to cool down

Fourth Transition Week

- Walk 5 minutes to warm up
- Run 5 minutes, walk 1 minute (Repeat 4 times)
- Walk 5 minutes to cool down

Fifth Transition Week

- Walk 5 minutes to warm up
- Run 5 minutes, walk 1 minute (Repeat 4 times)
- Walk 5 minutes to cool down

Sixth Transition Week

- Walk 5 minutes to warm up
- Run 7 minutes, walk 2 minutes (Repeat 3 times)
- Walk 5 minutes to cool down

Seventh Transition Week

- Walk 5 minutes to warm up
- Run 10 minutes, walk 3 minutes (Repeat 2 times)
- Walk 5 minutes to cool down

Eighth Transition Week

- Walk 5 minutes to warm up
- Run 12 minutes, walk 2 minutes (Repeat 2 times)
- Walk 5 minutes to cool down

Ninth Transition Week

- Walk 5 minutes to warm up
- Run 15 minutes, walk 2 minutes (Repeat 2 times)
- Walk 5 minutes to cool down

Tenth Transition Week

- Walk 5 minutes to warm up
- Run 20 minutes, walk 2 minutes (Repeat 2 times)
- Walk 5 minutes to cool down

Eleventh Transition Week

- Walk 5 minutes to warm up
- Run 30 minutes
- Walk 5 minutes to cool down

Twelfth Transition Week

- Walk 5 minutes to warm up
- Run 35 minutes
- Walk 5 minutes to cool down

HEALTHY EATING AND WEIGHT LOSS

It's Still Important to Eat Well Even Though You're No Longer Pregnant!

There is no doubt that all moms make sacrifices during pregnancy, avoiding certain foods and drinks for the benefit of our babies. And at some point, most of us moms have thought to ourselves, "I can't wait until my body is my own again," freeing us to return to some of the habits we gave up during pregnancy. Within a few weeks of becoming moms, we soon realize that while we are no longer housing and growing a baby, our bodies and our lives will truly never be our own, ever again! While I haven't met a mom yet who wasn't perfectly all right with leading a selfless existence, I do know this: With proper nutritional support, the joys of motherhood can far outweigh the challenges. On the flip side, poor nutritional habits will have that pregnancy glow fading faster than your ability to mentally recall anything that occurred before pregnancy (if you don't get that inside joke yet, just wait—you will!), and your energy sinking to an all-time low.

Proper food intake is a must for moms in the postnatal period—and not just those who are breastfeeding. It is vital that we come to terms with the fact that food is merely energy, and the better the choices we make in foods, the better our bodies can operate. When our bodies operate the way they were intended to, motherhood does not seem so taxing, and there will be plenty of energy to sustain you and your desire to live a purpose-filled life.

Healthy Snacks

Instead of heading down the path of poor snacking, opt out of the crash-and-burn effect and try some of these healthy snacks that are full of energy, packed with antioxidants, ready in a flash, and many of which are portable:

- Apple with a touch of peanut or almond butter
- Celery and peanut or almond butter
- Oatmeal with raisins or blueberries (it's not just for breakfast and is ready in 1 minute!)
- Vanilla or plain yogurt (opt for a lower-sugar version) with a handful of granola mixed in
- Fruit smoothie made with yogurt and frozen fruit
- Edamame
- Celery, carrots, and bell peppers with hummus
- Pita bread and hummus
- String cheese and whole-grain crackers
- High-fiber cereal and soy milk

Granted, you may not want to be snacking on edamame in the middle of the night, so don't forget that energy bars, such as Luna bars, may be an easier option given the time of day or night and your ability to prepare food. A time will come when you are able to prepare the foods you want to eat, but for now make sure you have foods on hand that need no preparation. Imagine yourself foraging for food with one free hand while the other cradles your baby (hence the handfuls of fish I ate!).

When you have the time and the energy, prepare some of the healthier options ahead of time and store them in individual containers in your refrigerator or pantry. This will help you have handy snacks on hand so that you can grab and go. If time or energy (or both) are not on your side, ask a relative or your spouse/partner to be your snack/meal assembly line for a day. Healing, feeding, and mothering takes energy, and energy is found in your food choices!

Research and real-life experience have taught me a lot about food and its ability to heal, prevent sickness, and sustain energy. It's time to put down the candy of your choice and treat your body as well as you did when you were pregnant. You'll be amazed at the result.

Food Is Energy

The biggest lesson to learn about food is this: It is simply an energy source as well as a way to prevent disease and ease the aches and pains associated with many ailments. It does not calm emotions and it does not mend a broken heart. Indulging in the wrong types of food does not solve any problems; in fact, it can make them bigger than they need to be. "Comfort" food is not really comforting; it is the memory associated with the food that is comforting. The next time you turn toward one of those comfort foods when life becomes a little more than you bargained for, stop yourself. Revert back to the memories associated with the food. Mentally revisit the person who prepared the dish, how he or she prepared it, and what special meaning or memory it has. Relish those memories, and you might just forget about eating the food after all.

One of the best ways to begin looking at food differently is to "interview" your food prior to consuming it. Here are three questions you should ask yourself about your food choices:

1. Can I eat this food every day and improve my health?
2. Is this food a source of good, clean energy?
3. Can this food lower my risk of disease and/or illness?

If the answer to any of the above questions is no, don't eat the food. It's just that simple. Good energy and good health come from good choices.

Your Main Source of Fuel: Carbohydrates

Carbohydrates, a nutrient source, are the body's main source of fuel. While protein and fats do provide fuel for life, the energy found in carbohydrates is broken down and available much sooner than other nutrient sources. Carbohydrates are typically broken down into two types—fast-acting (or simple carbohydrates) and slow-release (or complex carbohydrates).

Fast-Acting Carbs

Fast-acting carbohydrates will boost your energy levels quickly, but be aware that as quick as the energy comes, it also goes. Oftentimes, symptoms such as headaches, fatigue, memory loss, weight gain, mood swings, and hunger can be the result of overconsumption of fast-acting carbohydrates. However, you can alleviate these by choosing "positive" fast-acting carbs, rather than negative ones. Examples of negative fast-acting carbs are: white bread; Swedish fish; jelly beans; sugary, low-fiber cereals; baked goods made with white flour; and sodas. These simple sugars, highly refined foods, fatty foods, and junk food can provide energy, but they also come chock full of things your body does not need and has to spend energy breaking down and removing. Why waste energy removing something your body doesn't need or want?

Instead, choose a fast-acting carbohydrate like fruit. There is little to no prep time necessary, and not only is it packed with energy, but also fiber and antioxidants. The carbohydrates found in fruit happen to be the ones your body breaks down the fastest; therefore it is the quickest form of fuel. Fruits are also packed with water, and hydration is key to maintaining good energy.

Complex Carbs

Complex carbohydrates offer a more long-term energy supply. Foods that are packed with energy and are considered complex carbohydrates (meaning they take longer to be broken down by the body and therefore provide a more sustained energy boost) are oatmeal, whole-grain breads and pastas, beans, peas, lentils, root vegetables, brown rice, carrots, sweet potatoes, spinach, soybeans, soymilk, and yogurt, to name a few.

Since you're probably not going to memorize a list of complex versus simple carbohydrates; remember it like this: Carbohydrates that are filled with fiber or accompanied by lean protein and/or healthy fats will have a longer burn time, giving you energy for hours, not minutes, after consumption. Healthy proteins such as turkey, chicken, shellfish, and lean beef contain an amino acid called tyrosine, which stimulates the brain and increases alertness, and are all good options to accompany healthy carbs and slow down their absorption rate.

The Danger of a Postpartum Low-Carb Diet

Just as eating foods too high in carbohydrates will have you crashing and burning, so will diets that are low in carbohydrates. Most doctors do not recommended that new moms participate in low-carbohydrate diets while nursing or healing from surgery; check with your physician if you think your situation might be different. Remember that food is your source of energy for all functions, both those that care for your own body and those that care for your child's. Not only can a low-carbohydrate diet possibly reduce your milk production, slow your body's healing process, and leave you down in the dumps, it can also make it harder to lose weight! Carbohydrates not only aid in the mobilization of fat for fuel, but they also give you the energy for exercise. Extreme limiting of carbohydrates can also cause an energy deficit that stresses out the body, causing you to have food cravings and give in to them. Every cell in your body needs carbohydrates; do not fear nor shun them!

Iron

If you have a good mix of complex carbohydrates in your diet, are eating the recommended number of calories for your age and activity levels, and are still on the low-energy side of the equation, give consideration to your iron levels. According to *Energy-Boosting Foods* by nutritionist Susan Burke, low iron can cause your cells to have lower-than-adequate levels of oxygen, which can lead to inefficient use of carbohydrates, all of which translates to feelings of exhaustion. In this case, eating lean red meat on occasion can raise your iron levels. If symptoms continue, discuss it with your physician.

Foods That Heal

Many foods can speed recovery and provide energy all at the same time. Moms are queens of multitasking, and it is important that the foods we consume are as well.

With many layers of abdominal tissue being aggravated by surgery, inflammation is typical and can last for weeks following your baby's birth. Any tissue that has been cut will swell as part of the natural healing process. Once your body recognizes a wound, it sends blood cells and immune cells directly to the site, causing swelling, redness, heat, and sensations of stretching and pain. While medications can help reduce inflammation, therefore alleviating sensations, certain foods also contain anti-inflammatory properties and should be a part of our diets whenever possible.

The following is a list of foods that should be a part of our diets but are especially important in the first few months following a C-section.

- **Omega-3 essential fatty acids,** such as those found in walnuts, flaxseeds, pumpkin seeds, canola oils, and cold-water oily fish such as salmon or herring, have proven to be powerful anti-inflammatory agents. Some oils, such as olive, grape seed, and walnut, also contain inflammation-reducing properties.
- **Protein** is a must for tissues that are trying to repair themselves as they provide the amino acid building blocks that the body is not capable of producing itself. While some sources of protein (fatty red meats) can actually increase inflammation, other options, such as tofu, soy, and soymilk, are choices that can reduce swelling and the pain associated with it. If eating red meat, choose the leanest cuts possible, such as venison, and aim for grass-fed beef.
- Many herbs and foods such as **turmeric, oregano, basil, garlic, lemongrass, green tea, blueberries, and ginger** can be helpful in reducing inflammation. Both ginger and garlic also boost immunity and therefore are an important addition to your diet. Foods that are high in vitamin C have also been shown to improve collagen production and reduce further breakdown of collagen (a type of fiber

found within connective tissues) as well as assisting in the repair of other connective tissues and cartilage. Outside of oranges, there are many other foods that contain powerful amounts of vitamin C. It is very beneficial to keep a steady stream of vitamin C coming in all day long since it is not a vitamin that our bodies can make or store. Choose from kiwi, cantaloupe, mango, broccoli, red and yellow bell peppers, and potatoes to add variety to your diet and increase your vitamin C intake. Other additions to our diets to promote healing and connective tissue repair are eggs, garlic, strawberries, raspberries, and cranberries.

While it is a good idea to include these items in our diets, it is also important to avoid those that can add to our discomfort and fuel the swelling. Foods that have been known to increase inflammation are chocolate, coffee, dairy products, corn, peanuts, tomatoes, and wheat.

It is also important to increase your daily intake of water as it aids the body in toxin removal, which in turn can reduce swelling.

One last tip for gaining energy from healthy food sources is to include members of the B vitamin family whenever possible. Foods such as potatoes, lentils, beans, bananas, and tempeh, all of which are filled with B vitamins, actually help to unlock the energy in foods.

Foods That Protect and Preserve

We each have an internal coat of armor. If you are not careful, the armor will rust and weaken, but with a proper diet, you can be polishing your coat of armor daily. The earlier suggestion to interview food might seem quite silly, but it is actually exactly what you should be doing each and every time you reach for nourishment.

Our country has gone decades without taking food seriously. All we have to do is to watch a show such as *The Biggest Loser* to see how badly the wrong food choices can affect us, physically, mentally, and spiritually. Review the following list of foods and the diseases/conditions that they prevent or slow down the progression of. With this list in your hands at the grocery store, the right choice becomes an easy one to make.

- **Almonds:** heart disease, colon cancer
- **Apples:** heart disease, cancer, stroke
- **Avocado:** heart disease, cataracts, hardening of the arteries
- **Bell peppers:** go for the red, orange, or yellow variety, which are packed with vitamin C and therefore help to fight off the common cold as well as many forms of cancer
- **Blueberries:** can reverse or slow memory loss, and may reduce the risk of breast cancer
- **Broccoli:** cancer, heart disease
- **Cherries:** tumors, Alzheimer's disease
- **Flaxseed:** heart disease, stroke, depression, cancer
- **Garlic:** cancer, heart disease
- **Ginger:** cancer
- **Oatmeal:** heart disease, obesity
- **Olive oil:** heart attack, lowers blood pressure in women
- **Onions:** cancer
- **Oranges:** heart disease, inflammation
- **Pumpkin:** cancer
- **Salmon:** heart attack, heart diseases, Alzheimer's, dementia
- **Soy:** heart attack, may reduce the risk of cancer
- **Sweet potatoes:** cancer
- **Tea (black or green):** osteoporosis, cancer, heart attack

- **Tomatoes:** heart attack, cancer
- **Walnuts:** heart disease
- **Watermelon:** heart disease, cancer

Eating Well Doesn't Cost a Fortune!

Some people think that eating fresh, healthy food costs more, but that's not true. It does not always cost more; in fact, it can save you money and time. Recently I tested three fast-food drive thrus to see how much time and money I spent ordering food that seemed fast and cheap. I spent an average of 18 minutes (all three failed to get my order correct the first time, though) and $4.58 eating the not-so-healthy (but we think they are the healthier choice at a fast-food place) foods. At home, in all of five minutes, I can prepare a salmon burger (from frozen to ready to eat) on a whole-wheat bun, a small salad filled with veggies and topped with olive oil and balsamic vinaigrette, and a sweet potato that I cooked in the microwave for five minutes and then topped with cinnamon and Splenda. Not only was the homemade meal faster, filled with omega-3s, and rich in antioxidants, but it was also 150 calories less than the grilled chicken sandwich, potato, and drink from the drive thru—and under $5.

The same care and concern that you will put into feeding your baby as he/she begins to eat solid foods is the same care and concern that should go into your diet. After all, for the next 18 years (or more), your child's health and well-being is dependent on yours!

Counting Calories

Now that you know what to eat, the question remains how much to eat? Keep in mind that both breastfeeding and healing from surgery use energy, and energy for the body comes in the form of calories. Restricting your caloric intake during the first six weeks post-C-section can interfere with both. New moms should not worry about weight loss during this time. Instead, focus on eating as healthy as possible so that both your and your baby's immune systems can function well and so that you have the energy you need for your new full-time, 24-hour-a-day, seven-day-a-week job. After the initial recovery process, you can begin to change your caloric intake and expenditure levels in a moderate way to encourage returning to a healthy weight and reclaiming your body.

MOM to MOM: SHARE HEALTHY RECIPES!

The hardest part for me was the eating. I knew I was supposed to eat healthier, but what and how much? A one-hour consultation with a nutritionist set me on the right path. I then knew the amount of foods to eat and the foods that were best for me. Once I started asking friends for quick and healthy recipes or suggestions (I only asked friends who I knew ate the way they should) eating healthy became even easier! ~Seema

No two moms are alike, and their caloric needs vary as well. The following is the Harris Benedict Formula, which takes into consideration your daily activity levels and suggests an appropriate number of calories to *maintain* your current weight. (Nursing mothers need additional calories; look for those recommendations on the next page.) To lose weight, we need to take in fewer calories than suggested by the chart and burn off additional calories through exercise.

First, calculate your basal metabolic rate (BMR, the number of calories your body needs per day when at rest) using the following:

$$655 + (4.35 \times \text{weight in pounds}) + (4.7 \times \text{height in inches}) - (4.7 \times \text{age})$$

To determine your total daily calorie needs, multiply your BMR by the appropriate activity factor, as follows:

1. **If you are sedentary** (little or no exercise): Caloric Needs = BMR × 1.2

2. **If you are lightly active** (light exercise/sports 1 to 3 days/week): Caloric Needs = BMR × 1.375

3. **If you are moderately active** (moderate exercise/sports 3 to 5 days/week): Caloric Needs = BMR × 1.55

4. **If you are very active** (hard exercise/sports 6 to 7 days a week): Caloric Needs = BMR × 1.725

5. **If you are extra active** (very hard exercise/sports and/or physical job): Caloric Needs = BMR × 1.9

(Note: BMI Calculator: Harris Benedict Equation, n.d.)

Doctors recommend that nursing moms take in an additional 500 calories per day and drink a total of 80 to 96 ounces of fluid per day, not including additional fluid replacement postexercise.

Consider meeting with a nutritionist or dietitian no matter where you are in your pregnancy or recovery. Not only can a professional zero in on the right number of calories for you, but he or she can also look over your current diet and make recommendations that don't require drastic measures—which typically end in failure. A nutritionist or dietitian will also make recommendations for the types and amounts of important minerals and nutrients for your body during the pre- and postnatal stages.

Keys to Successful Weight Loss

As you think about your overall nutrition, you probably cannot avoid thinking about losing weight. After all, you have a burning desire to look and feel like your old self. Part of making this desire come to fruition means weight loss. Besides the health reasons, most women really do care how we look as well as how we feel. Along with losing the pounds will come tremendous gains in energy and health, if the right approach is taken. Again, do not consider weight loss until you have discussed your specific condition with your doctor.

For those who are "done" having children, this journey becomes about getting to a healthy weight and then staying there. For those who will have more children, this becomes a strategy for weight loss, a way to not gain more than the recommended amount of weight for the next pregnancy(ies), and a way to lose the baby weight again, and perhaps again. One thing is for certain: The body learns by repetition. Not only are you better at being pregnant each time around, but also with the proper strategy in place you will get better at losing the weight. Trust me—I have lost 50 pounds three times in my life, and each time it got easier!

Here are a few things of note when it comes to losing weight:

- Safe weight loss is one or two pounds per week. More than this can result in too severe of a change for the body, and the body can react by gaining all the weight back and then some.
- Low-carbohydrate diets often impede weight loss, and the initial weight loss experience on these diets is often fluid, not fat.
- 3,600 calories equals a pound. To lose weight, you must expend more calories per day than you consume, creating a caloric deficit.
- It is not ever recommended that adults limit their calorie intake per day to less than 1,200 calories (unless specified by their doctor).
- Nursing mothers often utilize an additional 300 to 500 calories a day to produce breast milk and should seek a nutritionist's advice on the correct number of calories to consume daily. Too few calories and too much exercise too soon will impair your milk production, so think about your priorities and eat and exercise accordingly. (You have the

rest of your life to diet and exercise, but you have only a few precious months to personally deliver a strong immune system and proper nutrition to your baby.)

- Eating too little will slow your metabolism, which in turn slows the weight loss process.

Overcoming Excuses and Fears

A key to incorporating a successful weight loss program into your lifestyle is overcoming the obstacles preventing your success. Once you begin to address them, you begin a journey that is about far more than weight loss. It's about a sense of confidence, purpose, and personal satisfaction, all of which lead to being a better mom—today and tomorrow. If you are having difficulty staying consistent with any of the three components we'll talk about next, ask yourself the following questions:

1. What is my ultimate goal?
2. How will accomplishing this goal affect the other areas of my life (for example, health, family, relationships, quality of life, and so on)?
3. Why is accomplishing this goal important to me?
4. What reasons do I give for not staying consistent or for holding back?

Human behavior is rooted in what we believe. Your feelings, thoughts, words, and actions are responses to and expressions of what you believe. Behavior is more than just what you do. It consists of four basic elements: what you feel, what you think, what you say, and what you do. These are also your personal power zones, meaning the areas through which you exercise your ability to choose. What you choose is a reflection of what you believe. We're often unaware of our underlying belief, however. If our behavior gets challenged, we use our thoughts and feelings to justify our behavior, successfully reinforcing whatever our belief is—or, we choose to take advantage of this opportunity to make a change.

Reasons that keep you from accomplishing life-giving goals are more accurately called "excuses." These "reasons" or "excuses" can be valuable to you, however, because they are indicators of what you believe. You have to be able to weigh whether or not a belief is encouraging you toward accomplishing your goals or keeping you from them. The questions provided are designed to cause the belief that primarily resides in your subconscious mind to come to your consciousness. Often the reasons you give are excuses to protect yourself, to cover fears you have, and to uphold whatever belief you have about yourself.

Mothers, out of our strong desire to nurture, tend to put meeting everyone else's needs before meeting our own. Unfortunately, that often leaves us exhausted, exasperated, and feeling that we aren't deserving of the same nurturing we give others in our lives. We feel selfish if we take time for ourselves. Women often describe feeling self-conscious after having a baby, particularly a C-section, due to the trauma to our body and our mind—the physical scar and hormonal surges become symbolic of an internal wound to our perception of who we are or how we're to be. One definition of the word trauma is simply "change." We don't believe we're able to overcome these changes and therefore isolate ourselves, comforting ourselves with food or by busying ourselves taking care of others.

The reality is that having a baby changes things—your body, your daily routine, and even your priorities. Remember, though, that your overall health and well-being are key to the health and well-being of your baby and your family. If you can recognize an excuse, you can decide whether or not you want to continue to allow that belief to remain. You can exercise your power to choose.

Three-Pronged Weight Loss Plan

From both personal experience and years of helping hundreds of clients through the weight loss journey, I have found that the most successful weight loss programs are those that incorporate all three of the following components:

- Cardiovascular conditioning
- Weight/resistance training
- Appropriate calorie intake

When all three of these components are fully embraced and put into practice on a consistent basis, the results are not only amazing but they are also *sustainable*. Also, from personal and professional experience, I know that most of us are willing to embrace one or two of the components and believe we can achieve our goals while still holding back on one of these fronts. Yes, implementing two of the three is much better than none of them, but the results will be limited and could be short term. If you are committed on one or two of the necessary fronts but holding back on the third, it is important to ask yourself the following questions:

1. Do I believe that change can happen?
2. Do I believe in myself?
3. Do I believe I can be successful and reach my goals?
4. Do I deserve to reach my goals?
5. Why am I holding back?

Once you have faced the reasons why you are holding back (discussed earlier) and begin to address them, then you will be able to connect on all fronts, leave your fears behind, and embark on a journey that becomes about far more than weight loss. It becomes about gaining self-esteem, self-love, self-belief, self-control, and self-appreciation, all of which will make us better moms today and tomorrow.

Cardiovascular Conditioning

Cardiovascular conditioning is important to weight loss because, when completed regularly and at the right effort level, it burns fat, reducing your weight. The exercises found in Chapter 5 will help you fulfill this aspect of the weight-loss plan.

MOM to MOM: FIND SUPPORT!

Until I fully engaged in cardio efforts, strength training, and healthy eating, it hadn't even really sunk in that I wasn't engaging in discovering the best version of myself. Change is hard. It is much easier to just let life keep going the way it is going then it is to stop and change direction. That is probably what held me back in prior attempts to live a healthier life. As a busy, working mom I felt that I was doing my part to take care of myself, but the truth is I wasn't. I always put my boys' and my husband's health before mine and often let the guilt of not wanting to take time for myself get in the way of my own well-being. Their health is hugely important to me, and so is spending quality time with them.

I do much better when those around me are on board and in recent months we have approached healthy living as a team. My husband and I are both fully engaged in our healthy routines, there to motivate each other to move, remind each other of things we should and shouldn't be eating, and hold each other accountable. It is working like a charm. Not only have we lost a lot of weight and many, many inches, but it has had a positive effect in every aspect of our lives and it is great to realize that we are great role models for our boys. My advice to other moms would be to find a loved one who is willing to work at changing habits with you, and then help each other daily. Eventually the healthier choices and the exercise becomes the only choice, but it can take a while to get there. In the meantime, having someone else involved is a huge help. In the end, I have found that healthy food doesn't take more time and with smart shopping, it isn't more expensive. As soon as I changed those beliefs and threw the excuses out the window the weight came off, and isn't ever coming back! ~Leah

Weight/Resistance Training

Weight training will increase the amount of lean muscle that you have, increasing the number of calories your body burns every minute of every day, and the proper caloric intake will create the caloric deficit necessary for losing weight. Weight training is vital to weight loss, because without the addition of lean muscle, we will still have to spend more hours than we care to performing cardiovascular exercise. Muscle tissue burns up to five times as many calories every minute of every day. Therefore, for every pound of lean muscle you add, you increase the pace at which you are losing weight.

No worries, ladies: We do not have enough testosterone in our bodies to bulk up. In fact, the addition of muscle along with the burning of subcutaneous fat makes us smaller! You may know, and I do too, women who had begun weight training and did get bigger instead of smaller. This is due to either a lack of reduction in calories or a lack of fat-burning cardiovascular exercise. The exercises in Chapter 6 will help you meet the goals of this aspect of the weight-loss plan.

Proper Caloric Intake

A caloric deficit created by reducing your food intake alone can not only leave you exhausted and crabby, but can also make it difficult to produce breast milk and heal from your surgery. Since one pound equals 3,600 calories, you would need to reduce your daily caloric intake by 500 calories to lose one pound of fat per week; to lose two pounds over a week you would need to reduce your daily intake by 1,000 calories. Such a drastic reduction of calories can negatively affect your body, so much so that your body may start to store fat instead of burn it, thinking that you are a cave woman!

Our DNA has not changed at the rate that our levels of civilization have. In fact, your body still expects there to be ample food supplies for only a few months out of the year. During those months of feasting, your body is on track to store up calories in the form of fat, which will then be burned to sustain you during the many months of famine (winter with less food availability). Your body also believes that you must expend energy to hunt and gather your food. (Little does it know that you can drive up to a window and be handed more food than you really need without lifting a finger!) This gap between our DNA and society makes it easy to gain weight and oftentimes difficult to lose it.

No One Prong Is Enough

Many believe that it takes willpower to lose weight, but all it really takes is knowledge and the ability, at times, to trick the body. Since you are programmed to store fat and programmed to believe that a sudden reduction of calories means a famine has set in, drastically reducing your food intake sends your body into hibernation mode. While in this mode, your body slows down your caloric burn rate (metabolism) so that you store fat and will be able to survive on that fat for as long as the famine may last. This is why losing weight by dieting alone not only makes you feel bad, but also doesn't actually work for long-term weight loss or maintenance. Since an abundance of food is just a phone call away, your mind will eventually take over, a giant pizza will land on your doorstep, and one piece will turn into five or six. Programmed to feast after the famine, you really don't have a fighting chance. You will give in and most likely end up gaining the weight back over the course of the feasting days, weeks, and months.

Reading this information should bring a sense of relief! It is not your fault! You are reacting the exact way you are programmed to react. Once you reprogram your mind through proper exertion and proper caloric intake, you will overcome the feast or famine reaction, lose and/or maintain the desired weight, and feel great. Caloric deficit from exercise alone will leave you little time for anything but exercise. Reducing your intake and increasing your activity levels will make weight loss seem not so fatiguing and difficult!

So dieting alone will not fix the problem. What would happen if we tried to lose the baby weight by performing cardiovascular exercise alone? Let's take that same 1,000-calorie reduction a day to lose two pounds a week for a total of 50 pounds lost. For example, knowing that I can burn four calories a minute from fat (this is me, not everyone), I would have to exercise for four hours and twenty minutes every day to lose the weight. I certainly cannot think of much that is more miserable than that! Not only would I be hating life by the end of the first week, but I would also have just about every injury in the book by the end of the third week. I would be crabby, burned out, and left hating exercise, and it would still take me six months to lose the weight. It's not worth it, and it's physically impossible.

By now you can see that losing weight by diet or cardiovascular exercise alone seems and is a miserable option. But, moderately reducing your caloric intake and increasing your activity levels every day lead to a much more sustainable routine that sheds the weight and has your body noticing nothing but good effects.

When you combine all three components you lose weight, drop clothing sizes, and operate your body more efficiently, leaving you with more energy than you will know what to do with!

EPILOGUE

It Takes a Village

Community can be the saving grace of motherhood. Most new moms feel isolated and alone in their struggles to be perfect moms and not lose themselves in the process. As birds of a feather flock together, so should moms. Surround yourself with other moms; share tears of joy and sadness in the company of those who have been there, are there, or are on their way to being there. There is no shame in any of the feelings a new mom (or seasoned veteran mom) experiences. You will most likely find that the mom you think has it all together because she seems perfect on the outside would really love a shoulder to cry on and a friend to help her through the tough times.

Community comes in many different forms today. It can be found in neighborhoods, schools, work places, exercise groups such as StrollerFit, playgroups such as StrollerFriends, and moms' groups both online and in person. Community can be found in social media, websites, blogs, phone calls, and coffee shops. With all the trials and tribulations of motherhood, know this: You are not alone! Seek out your own community and flourish in your strength, beauty, and ability to give and receive love and support! Here are some of my favorite websites:

- *www.revolution-fitness.com*
- *www.marybethknight.com*
- *www.strollerfit.com*
- *www.sparkpeople.com*
- *www.babyfit.com*
- *www.girlfriendology.com*

In addition, look for *Strategies for the C-Section Mom* on Facebook!
In health . . .

BIBLIOGRAPHY

Anderson, Steven J., Bernard A. Griesemer, Miriam D. Johnson, Thomas J. Martin, Larry G. McLain, Thomas W. Rowland, and Eric Small. "Medical Concerns in the Female Athlete." *Pediatrics,* September 2000: 610–13.

Anthony, Lenita. *Pre- and Post-Natal Fitness: A Guide for Fitness Professionals from the American Council on Exercise.* San Diego, CA: American Council on Exercise, 2002.

Antoniades, Spiro. 2009. Preventing Back Pain During Pregnancy. *http://health.discovery.com/centers/pregnancy/backpain.html* (accessed January 17, 2010).

www.befitmom.com/abdominal_seperation.html [sic] (accessed January 17, 2010).

Bonyata, Kelly. 2003. Exercise and Breastfeeding. *www.kellymom.com/health/lifestyle/mom-exercise.html* (accessed January 17, 2010).

Byrd, Andrea. 2002 Serotonin and Its Uses. *http://serendip.brynmawr.edu/bb/neuro/neuro99/web1/Byrd.html* (accessed August 2009).

Cerner Multum Inc. 2009. Morphine. *www.drugs.com/morphine*.html (accessed January 18, 2010).

Cowlin, Ann. *Women's Fitness Program Development*. Champaign, IL: Human Kinetics, 2002.

Cram, Catherine. *Prenatal & Postpartum Fitness*. Middleton, WI: Comprehensive Fitness Consulting, LLC, 2003.

Datta, Sanjay. *Obstetric Anesthesia Handbook, Fifth Edition*. New York, NY: Springer, LLC, 2010.

Diaz-Bordon, Carolina. 2007. 10 Energy Boosting Foods. *http:// dhf.ediets.com/news/NewsArticle.jsp?id=999999933* (accessed January 17, 2010).

Douglas, Ann. 2004. Cesarean Recovery: What Nobody Tells You. *http://pregnancyandbaby.sheknows.com/pregnancy/Detailed/Cesarean-recovery--What-nobody-tells-you-60.htm* (accessed January 17, 2010).

Easton, John. 2005. As Morphine Turns 200, Drug That Blocks Its Side Effects Reveals New Secrets. *www.uchospitals.edu/news/2005/20050519-morphine.html* (accessed January 17, 2010).

Gaither, Heather. 2007–2009. Your C-Section Recovery at Home. *www.the-essential-infant-resource-for-moms.com/C-Section-Recovery.html* (accessed January 18, 2010).

Harms, Roger W. 2007. Guide to a Healthy Pregnancy. *www .americanpregnancy.org/labornbirth/epidural.html* (accessed January 18, 2010).

HealthCheck Systems. 1997–2010. Understanding Your Body Fat Percentage. *www.healthchecksystems.com/bodyfat.htm* (accessed January 18, 2010).

Izzy, Minti.Com contributor. 2007. Tips to Make Recovery from Ceasarean Section Easier. *www.minti.com/parenting-advice/382/Tips-to-Make-Recovery-from-Ceasarean-Section-Easier/* (accessed January 17, 2010).

Jeffries, Melissa. How C-Sections Work. *http://health.howstuffworks. com/c-section.htm* (accessed January 17, 2010).

Jegtvig, Shereen. 2009. Anti–inflammatory Foods: Can the Foods You Eat Make a Difference in Chronic Pain? *http://nutrition.about.com/od/ dietsformedicaldisorders/a/antiinflamfood.htm* (accessed January 17, 2010).

Kantor, Gareth S. 2001. Ask an Expert: Spinal vs. Epidural for C-Section. *www.netwellness.org/question.cfm/22581.htm* (accessed January 18, 2010).

Karacabey, Kursat. 2008. Cesarean Section: Topic Overview. *www.webmd .com/baby/tc/cesarean-section-topic-overview (accessed January 18, 2010).*

Karacabey, Kursat, Ozcan Saygin, Recep Ozmerdivenli, Erdal Zorba, Ahment Godekermedan, and Vedat Bulut. "The Effects of Exercise on the Immune System and Stress Hormones in Sportswomen." *Neuroendocrinology Letters,* No. 4, Volume 26, August 2005.

Maffetone, Phillip. *The ABCs of Hormonal Stress.* Stamford, NY: David Barmore Productions, 1999.

Maffetone, Phillip. *Eating for Endurance.* Stamford, NY: David Barmore Productions, 1996.

Maleskey, Gale, Mary Kittel, and the Editors of *Prevention. The Hormone Connection.* Emmaus, PA: Rodale Inc., 2001.

Mayo Clinic Staff. 2008. Stress: Win Control over the Stress in Your Life. *www.mayoclinic.com/health/stress/SR00001* (accessed January 18, 2010).

Mayo Clinic Staff. 2009. C-Section—Overview: Why It's Done, Risks, What You Can Expect, and Recovery. www.mayoclinic.com/health/c-section/MY00214 (accessed January 18, 2010).

Men's Fitness Staff. "Energy-Boosting Foods: These 10 Foods Will Keep Your Motor Revving All Day and All Night." *Men's Fitness*, May 2003.

Murray, Jennifer. 2008. Good Carbs Versus Bad Carbs. *www.proteins-carb-fats .suite101.com/article.cfm/good_carbs_versus_bad_carbs#ixzz0cPFXGTLH (accessed January 18, 2010).*

Neifert, Marianne, R. *Dr. Mom's Guide to Breastfeeding.* New York: Penguin Group, 1998.

Pick, Marcelle. 2005. Reducing Inflammation: The Natural Approach. *www.womentowomen.com/inflammation/naturalantiinflammatories.aspx* (accessed January 18, 2010).

Porter, Colleen Kay. 1994. Strength Training for Moms. *www.afn .org/~cporter/strength* (accessed January 18, 2010).

Quinn, Elizabeth. 2006. The Q-Angle and Injuries in Women Athletes. *http://sportsmedicine.about.com/od/women/a/Q_angle.htm* (accessed January 18, 2010).

Quinn, Elizabeth. 2009. Proper Hydration for Exercise: Water or Sports Drinks? *http://sportsmedicine.about.com/od/hydrationandfluid/a/ ProperHydration.htm* (accessed January 18, 2010).

Reynolds, Gretchen. "How Exercise and Bed Rest in Pregnancy Can Co-Exist." *New York Times*, March 22, 2007.

Treuth, Margarita S., Nancy F. Butte, and Maurice Puyau. 2005. Pregnancy-Related Changes in Physical Activity, Fitness: Discussion. *www.medscape.com/viewarticle/504467_4* (accessed January 18, 2010).

Turner, John. 2009. Exercise in Pregnancy. *www.sportsmed.iu.edu/presentations/ExerciseInPregnancy_Public.PDF* (accessed January 18, 2010).

Washington State Department of Health, Office of Environmental Health, Safety, and Toxicology. 2009. Fish Facts for Healthy Nutrition. *www.doh.wa.gov/ehp/oehas/fish/fishfaq.htm* (accessed on January 18, 2010).

WebMD. "Kegel Exercises." *http://women.webmd.com/tc/kegel-exercises-topic-overview.* Accessed January 18, 2010.

Weiss, Robin Elise, et al. 1995–1999. The Cesarean Section FAQ. *www.childbirth.org/section/CSFAQ.html* (accessed January 18, 2010).

Woolston, Chris. "B Vitamins Don't Boost Energy Drinks' Power." *LA Times,* July 14, 2008.

INDEX

ABOUT THE AUTHOR

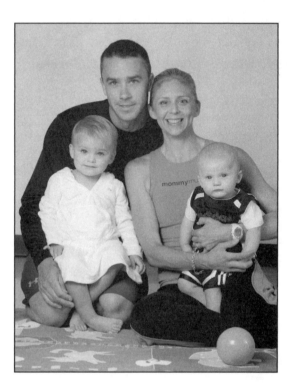

Mary Beth Knight is the creator of the restore the core®, restore the core power®, mommymuscle® sculpt, mommymuscle® c-section recovery workout, the mommymuscle® 8-week challenge, mommymuscle® mom 'n tot yoga program, and the Fit as Family exercise programs used throughout the StrollerFit® franchise organization. Since 1999, StrollerFit has provided moms with appropriate workouts for motherhood. The perfect blend of cardiovascular exercise mixed with strength training, StrollerFit allows moms to work out with their baby by their side! The exercise classes are also a great place for moms to find support, ask other moms for advice, and make lifelong friends—all while introducing their children to exercise and healthy habits at an early age. Children ages six weeks to six years love coming to StrollerFit classes as it provides a learning atmosphere and lots of laughs as the moms sing songs, count in foreign languages, and entertain their babies while on the move. For more information, or to find a class near you, visit *www.strollerfit.com* today.

Mary Beth is also the creator of the Muscle Bar®, a portable weighted bar and resistance tube combination that creates long, lean muscles, and the Fit Revolution 10-Week Weight-Loss Program®. As the maternal fitness expert for Discovery Health, Mary Beth answers questions from moms worldwide and offers her real-mom advice on a pregnancy and parenting blog that can be found at *www.inspire.com/groups/pregnancy-and-parenting/*. Along with her husband Eric, Mary Beth owns Revolution Fitness® (*www.revolution-fitness.com*) in Cincinnati, Ohio. Mary Beth's most important role is mom to Mazie and Miles!